Putting Patients Last

Putting Patients Last

How the NHS keeps the
ten commandments of business failure

Peter Davies & James Gubb

Civitas: Institute for the Study of Civil Society
London

First Published July 2009

© Civitas 2009
77 Great Peter Street
London SW1P 2EZ
Civitas is a registered charity (no. 1085494)
and a company limited by guarantee, registered in
England and Wales (no. 04023541)

email: books@civitas.org.uk

ISBN 978-1-906837-09-9

Independence: Civitas: Institute for the Study of Civil
Society is a registered educational charity (No. 1085494) and
a company limited by guarantee (No. 04023541). Civitas is
financed from a variety of private sources to avoid over-
reliance on any single or small group of donors.

All publications are independently refereed. All the Institute's
publications seek to further its objective of promoting the
advancement of learning. The views expressed are those of
the authors, not of the Institute.

Typeset by
Civitas

Printed in Great Britain by
The Cromwell Press Group
Trowbridge, Wiltshire

Contents

Authors

Dr Peter Davies BSc (Hons), MBChB (Leeds 1989), Diploma in Primary Health Care, FRCGP, is a GP Principal at Keighley Road Surgery, Illingworth, Halifax. He also serves as a GP appraiser for Calderdale PCT, is Chair of the Yorkshire Faculty of The Royal College of General Practitioners and is a Yorkshire Faculty Representative on the RCGP Council. He writes regularly for medical publications, including the *British Medical Journal* and the *British Journal of General Practice*. The views expressed in this publication are his own.

James Gubb is Director of the Health Unit at Civitas. After graduating in Philosophy, Politics and Economics from St John's College, Oxford, he worked briefly in criminal law, before joining Civitas in June 2006, where he has worked on European issues and health policy. His previous publications on health include *'Just how well are we?'*, *'Why are we waiting?'* and *'Checking-up on Doctors: a review of the Quality and Outcomes Framework'*. He is a regular contributor to print, broadcast and healthcare media.

Acknowledgements

We owe a great debt of gratitude to many people, not least everyone we have had the privilege of speaking to and working with over the past few months and, in some cases, years. Personal experiences aside, it is they who have more often than not provided the insight behind this book and kept our thinking on an even keel.

Among them, we are particularly grateful to those who have taken the time to read, digest and comment on our many drafts: Professor Robbie Foy, Dr Chris Johnstone, Dr Steve Chambers, Nick Seddon, Robert Whelan, Oliver Meller-Herbert, Katherine Lee and Laura Brereton. Their copy-editing, criticisms and at times brutal honesty have saved us many errors, inconsistencies and inappropriate turns of phrase. Not all will necessarily agree with our conclusions, but (hopefully) our arguments are more refined as a result of their input.

Abbreviations

BAMM	British Association of Medical Managers
BMA	British Medical Association
CHRE	Council for Healthcare Regulatory Excellence
CQC	Care Quality Commission
CQUIN	Commissioning for Quality and Innovation
DGH	District General Hospital
DH	Department of Health
FESC	Framework for Procuring External Support for Commissioners
FTs	Foundation Trusts
GMC	General Medical Council
GMS	General Medical Services
HPA	Health Protection Agency
ICO	Integrated Care Organisation
IHI	Institute for Healthcare Improvement
MMC	Modernising Medical Careers
NAO	National Audit Office
NHS	National Health Service
NICE	National Institute for Health and Clinical Excellence
NMC	Nursing and Midwifery Council
NPfIT	National Programme for Information Technology
NPSA	National Patient Safety Agency
PCT	Primary Care Trust
PMETB	Postgraduate Medical and Education Training Board
QOF	Quality and Outcomes Framework
SHA	Strategic Health Authority
VHA	Veterans Health Administration
WHO	World Health Organisation

Foreword

I recently heard from Dr Peter Davies and Mr James Gubb, members of Civitas and linked closely to its health unit, requesting that I write a brief foreword in this publication on the elements of my book on business failure.

As a citizen of the US without in-depth knowledge of the issues confronting the National Health Service, my brief comments only deal with the almost fatal traps that stand in the way of organisations, individuals and nations. Let me make it clear that the national debate on health care is a major current issue in the US as well.

The simple fact is that 'success' is a dangerous word and is a journey—not a destination. And, on that journey there is constant danger. Because the subject of this book is health care, let me suggest that there are two dangerous viruses ready to explode in any organisation's leadership. The minute that individuals and organisations begin to really believe they have reached the goal of success, these viruses emerge. They are arrogance and complacency.

The 'Ten Commandments' of my book deal with the symptoms and the results of these viruses breaking loose. If Dr Davies and Mr Gubb find that they can translate some of these Commandments into a valid discussion involving the National Health Service, it would seem to me that would be a worthwhile effort.

One doesn't know how to avoid failure unless one recognises it. Remember that the important thing is the journey. And, if any journey must be successful, it would be that dealing with the health of a nation.

Donald Keough
Author, 'The Ten Commandments for Business Failure'
Past President and CEO, the Coca Cola Company

Preface

The inspiration for this volume comes from an unlikely source so far as health care is concerned: the past president and CEO of the Coca-Cola Company, Donald R. Keough, and his authoritative book *The Ten Commandments for Business Failure*—a tale of ten blunders that he and many others have 'witnessed companies and individuals making time and time again that so consistently lead to failure they should be written in stone'.

To apply Keough's ten commandments to health care— and particularly the National Health Service in England— will, we know, be controversial. The NHS, as a whole, is not a business; and certainly not a multinational corporation. However, recent reforms have unquestionably sought to stimulate competition between healthcare providers and increase the choices available to patients. Though still part of a single-payer (tax-funded) structure, NHS *organisations* in both primary and secondary care are now cast very much as semi-autonomous businesses and faced with business-like incentives.[a]

(a) We would like to make a point about vocabulary at this juncture. In this book we speak of the NHS as a business or collection of businesses, following the line that has typically been taken either implicitly or explicitly by government policy since the publication of the Griffiths Report in 1983. As we acknowledge in the introduction, the NHS is not a business in the sense in which economists normally understand the term. However, to write 'business' thus, using inverted commas to indicate ironic or incorrect usage, would be, in a work of this length, a tedious affectation. We therefore ask the reader to understand that the term is used here in the sense in which health policy-makers in Whitehall currently deploy it.

Of equal importance, we would argue that Keough's book is not just concerned with business, but with service. None of his commandments centre overtly on finance, structure or procedure. Instead they are concerned with the underlying culture, emotion and politics that make successful organisations tick and that enable them to maintain a resolute focus on the people they serve (customers or patients).

In truth, we found it almost uncanny in reading Keough's commandments how many times both of us, independently, sat back and thought 'the NHS does this—a lot'. In essence, it focused our minds on the roots of the NHS's current problems. No-one can say there has been a lack of effort in trying to make the system work over the past decade or so: the frenetic pace of change has, at times, been frightening. Structures and processes have been organised, re-organised and re-disorganised; and it's almost certain they are still far from being right.

Lost in all this, however, have been people: patients, doctors, nurses, health professionals and, yes, even the much-maligned managers. Patients, the customers of fledgling businesses in the NHS, should be the focus of everything these organisations do. And, in a labour-intensive industry like healthcare, people are *the* resource by which this can be achieved.

Yet, with so much attention having been diverted to changing structures and satisfying seemingly endless central initiatives, targets and regulation, energies have shifted elsewhere. Patient care has far too often been relegated to second, third, or even fourth place after the government, the Department of Health, strategic health authorities and numerous regulators have been satisfied. It's not that staff have stopped caring, but that poor practice has either become ingrained to the extent that it's difficult to see things differently; or that staff prefer to acquiesce because they've tried so many times to change the system and got nowhere.

There's a brilliant passage in Keough's book that we would like to share with you here:

> It's so easy to lose sight of the customer [read patient], to think dispassionately about an amorphous mass called the market or market segment.
>
> There are, except as statistical abstractions, no such things as market segments. There are only people. They have faces. Visualise your audience. Visualise specific people and think hard about just what you're going to do for them that day.[1]

It is time, in our view, for the NHS—and the organisations that make it up—to start backing people rather than processes. It is time for the government to stop over-estimating the importance of legislation, crude measurement and regulation as markers of success and put faith in the power of frontline organisations to drive quality. Effective regulation is important, but the autonomy associated with a more business-like framework means nothing if all it is used for is finding more innovative ways of meeting central targets.

We should say two things at this point, however. First, this book is not a policy prescription, and does not claim to have all the answers to the problems it describes (though we hope some of our suggestions are useful). Second, we fully recognise that in applying Keough's commandments we will no doubt be accused of fitting evidence to our case. We are, strange though it may sound, relatively comfortable with this. Of course, we believe our diagnosis is accurate and that we have provided sufficient evidence to show it to be so. But, more importantly, our aim—one of us a doctor, one a health researcher—is twofold. First, to attempt to bridge the gap that both of us perceive between policy-making and the day-to-day practice of medicine, which has widened to a chasm in recent years. And second, to provoke a debate; a discussion, if you like, about all those things that so many in the NHS are saying to us in private, yet so few are saying in public.

We welcome you to join us.

Peter Davies
James Gubb

Introduction

For many years now the National Health Service (NHS) in England has been encouraged to think about itself, and its activities, in business terms. Providers of NHS services must compete for custom to survive, patients are consumers, and for the government the 'science' of performance management and target-setting has ruled the roost. The contrast to earlier models of service is marked. In these, the role of government was, in the words of the NHS's architect Nye Bevan, restricted to '[providing] the medical profession with the best and most modern apparatus of medicine'.[1] Quality was 'guaranteed' by professional standards, rather than the state and/or markets.

The shift of thinking from one school to the other developed in the Thatcher years and is most clearly seen in the establishment of the internal market and purchaser/provider split. 'The NHS', documents health policy analyst Rudolf Klein, 'was to mimic those characteristics of the market that would promote greater efficiency within the framework of a public service committed to distributing access to resources according to need.'[2] After flirting with the idea of partnership and a 'third way', New Labour bought into the same vision, sharpening incentives and developing the range and scope of the market through patient choice, 'world-class commissioning' and payment-by-results in particular. As Simon Stevens, a former health adviser to Tony Blair, said of the choice policy: if NHS organisations aren't efficient enough to perform the operations there will be 'a bunch of Germans [aka private providers] coming round the corner that will'.[3] Many NHS organisations, particularly foundation trusts, are now as much businesses as they are public bodies.

The jury is still out on the use of such market mechanisms in a single-payer (tax-funded) health system like the NHS.

1

The emphasis it places on financial discipline, innovation and being responsive to patients is welcome, but there are many consequences that give cause for concern—not least possible bankruptcies and, crucially, the impact of many confused and conflicting incentives on the culture of medicine and nursing that is so vital to quality of care. Reform has produced market forces, yet rigid rules ensure that competition is more often between primary and secondary care than aligned to the experience and needs of patients; and while government rhetoric is for NHS organisations to look out to communities, it continues to micromanage the service like never before.[4] As the economist John Kay has argued—and this is a theme that runs through this book—effective market economies are embedded in an elaborate social, political and cultural context; a context that is underdeveloped where the NHS is concerned.[5]

That said, if the NHS is to operate under such business and market-like terms, then it is fair to ask how good a business—or collection of businesses—the NHS currently is. In 2008, the former president of the Coca-Cola Company, Donald R. Keough published an influential book on success in this field, *The Ten Commandments of Business Failure*.[6] In it he draws on years of experience to argue that any step-by-step plan offering 'tried and true advice' in business will inevitably lead to huge disappointment; there are no sets of rules or formulas that will guarantee success. However, what he does offer are sure-fire ways to fail. His 'ten commandments for business failure' are blunders that he and many other successful businessmen who have accredited the book have witnessed companies and individuals making time and time again that 'so consistently lead to failure they should be written in stone'. They quit taking risks; are inflexible; isolate themselves; assume infallibility; play the game close to the foul line; don't take time to think; put their faith in experts and outside consultants; love bureaucracy; send mixed messages; are afraid of the future. Staff, as a result, lose passion for work. What is notable is that none of the commandments focus overtly on finance, structure or procedure; they cut much deeper, concerned with the underlying culture, emotion and politics that make successful businesses work. Without due attention to this, they—and, for that matter, most organisations—will forever underachieve.

Though there are nuances particular to each commandment, and exceptions to every rule, we contend that large swathes of the NHS are currently following all ten of them. For the new business-focused and market-driven NHS to work, organisations must have the freedom to concentrate their energies on delivering the best possible service to each and every patient. Mirroring experience in other sectors, successful providers and commissioners will be those who assess, listen to and respond to patient needs, and split their customers into different profiles for whom they will offer different, personalised, services.[7] They will also be those who fully embrace the need not just for structural change, but more importantly for cultural change that embeds quality improvement and puts patients, rather than the government or the profession, first. This has yet to happen. Instead, under pressure from hotchpotch and inconsistent reform, the worst types of business (and public service) are emerging in this brave new world: those that are risk-averse and obsessed with internal processes, bureaucracy and fads; businesses that dance to the tune of their shareholders and boards of directors (in this case the government, Department of Health and NHS Executive), rather than focusing on customers (patients) and what they need.

This is not to portray NHS organisations as ineffectual cousins of the private sector. For one thing, many private sector companies fall into the same trap, thinking first about meeting their shareholders' needs and investing in large reconfigurations to meet performance targets. These are the companies—think Woolworths, Little Chef and General Motors—that have now gone to the wall or are struggling. Second, many of the problems in NHS organisations are likely to be systemic and cultural, rather than the result of individual error or lack of foresight. Organisations are still judged less by how effectively they treat patients, and more by performance against central priorities and standards.[a]

The wider point is this: so long as the government continues to over-estimate the importance of legislation and regulation as markers of success, and under-estimate the power of the businesses it has created to transform healthcare delivery, the NHS will continue to flounder. As Keough's ten commandments emphasise, successful business and noteworthy change very rarely come about through command-and-control or following nicely packaged toolkits. Instead, they come about through hard work, clarity of vision and an organisational focus on those factors so often talked about but so rarely addressed: leadership, teamwork, communication, flexibility, relationship-building, honesty, humanity, trust, and the occasional bit of peer pressure. It is this that we wish to stress. Currently in the NHS we have the extra costs of business and competitive

---

(a) For an example of this, we need look no further than Mid Staffordshire NHS Foundation Trust, which was rated as 'good' on quality of service by the Healthcare Commission in 2008 despite running a standardised mortality rate significantly higher than comparable hospitals.

processes minus the benefits that could be delivered if organisational autonomy were genuine and competition real.[8] Without a change of emphasis in the long-term (in more than just rhetoric), without due attention to the social, cultural and political context that supports successful business, our fear is this will only get worse. The consequences of this—particularly with the NHS's budget likely to see real-term cuts in the next few years[9]—are many, causing harm to patients, staff, managers and politicians; while inevitably increasing the cost to taxpayers. If we do not want yet another reassertion of central control and pointless reorganisation of services, the learning must start now.

NHS plc

The applicability of our premise, of analysing the NHS as a business or collection of businesses, may of course be questioned. The NHS is not a business in the strict sense of the word. It cannot go bankrupt (unless the state does) and is neither privately owned, nor run for profit; it is publicly owned and exists to provide a public service. However, since the publication of the Griffiths Report in 1983 the organisations *that make it up*—and provide frontline services —have been increasingly cast as businesses that must 'look after customers'. Post-Griffiths, the whole of government policy can be seen as a search for the levers that would encourage such a focus.[1] The 'internal', 'quasi' or 'mimic' market solution settled on in 2002 is both the latest and most far-reaching: organisations—at least those on the provider side—are more than just businesses in rhetoric.[2]

At the systemic level, starting with the Secretary of State for Health, an organisational hierarchy pervades the NHS, running through the Department of Health (which has its own board), the NHS Chief Executive (David Nicholson) and regional Strategic Health Authorities (SHAs) to Primary Care Trusts (PCTs), general practice, community organisations and NHS trusts. Emanating from the Department of Health (DH) is a keen focus on finance, 'profit' (or generating surplus) and management strategy. Each year the Operating Framework sets out an overview of priorities for the NHS; and each quarter the NHS publishes an update from David Flory, Director General for NHS Finance, Performance and Operations, that outlines the NHS's financial position, as well as progress against the framework. The DH also has its own Commercial Directorate that 'functions as the central point in securing best value as well as achieving greater levels of effectiveness for the DH and the NHS through the use of best commercial practices and better commercial relationships'.[3] SHAs and the foundation trust regulator, Monitor, have the power to intervene if NHS trusts/foundation trusts[(a)] do not demonstrate continued financial and managerial competence.[b][4]

Beneath such overarching bodies, the NHS functions as a market, with a split between geographically-based 'commissioners' or purchasers of care—the local PCTs—and service providers, including NHS trusts, foundation trusts, general practice, community services, and the independent and voluntary sectors. The rationale for this split is a business one: to improve technical and allocative efficiency by 'encouraging providers to respond more accurately and effectively to the needs of individual patients in order to retain contracts'.[5]

In performing their function (dubbed 'world class commissioning') PCTs are tasked to do much more than just contract management. They aim to deliver a more strategic and long-term approach to commissioning services, with a clear focus on need and delivering improved health outcomes. They are inspected on their use of resources and expected to drive value in the system by using financial leverage to commission more effective services, the 'adding life to years and years to life' of the world-class com-

---

(a) Foundation trusts are (groups of) hospitals providing secondary care in the NHS. They still operate as NHS bodies, but are free from direct line management by the DH and SHAs, with legal status as independent public benefit corporations. Foundation trusts can retain their surpluses and borrow to invest in new and improved services. They are accountable to their local communities through their members and governors, to their commissioners through contracts, to Parliament, and to Monitor as their regulator.

(b) Monitor also actively encourages training programmes and business management strategies such as service-line reporting.

missioning agenda. One of the competencies against which they are assessed is their ability to 'stimulate the market'.[6]

Providers, for their part, are cast as businesses and are supposed to have 'embraced the idea that the customer is king'.[7] While hospital trusts have always had a statutory duty to break even and ensure they are financially viable, it is now pivotal. Financial incentives have been sharpened considerably in recent years. For one thing, financial viability and sustainability is crucial to achieving, and maintaining, the additional freedoms associated with foundation trust status. More widely, a trust's income is dependent on its ability to compete for business. Patients have a choice of hospital and the payment-by-results system ensures the hospital that a patient chooses gets paid for treating them (i.e. per case), rather than by block contract.[8] Quality, as well as being about clinical outcomes and safety, is increasingly cast as care that is personal to each individual.[9] Key to the 'informed' exercise of choice, then, are indicators of patient satisfaction, information at websites such as NHS Choices and Dr Foster, and the annual ratings given to trusts by the Healthcare Commission watchdog, to which quality of care and how well a trust uses its resources contributes heavily.[c] In such an environment there will inevitably be winners and losers, so a Cooperation and Competition Panel has been set up to pick up on anti-competitive practice, and the DH is currently consulting on a failure regime.[10] [d]

(c) As of April 2009, the Healthcare Commission was subsumed into the Care Quality Commission (CQC), along with the Mental Health Commission and the Commission for Social Care Inspection. As this book went to print the CQC was still developing its inspection regime.

(d) Additional plans are now being introduced to make a proportion of secondary care providers' income conditional on quality and

Similar moves are afoot in primary care. While general practice has been run on a small business model since well before the start of the NHS, there has been a renewed attention to profitability since the introduction of the substantial pay-for-performance element of the new GMS contract (the Quality and Outcomes Framework or QOF).[11] Lord Darzi's review of the NHS in 2008 also seeks an additional competitive impulse by introducing a series of polyclinics (or GP-led health centres)[(e)] and giving patients greater choice of GP practice. Before the end of 2007, only a small number of PCTs had used competitive tendering for primary care services, but a year later more than 100 practices were being run by alternative providers—GP-led companies, corporate providers and social enterprises.[12] There are also efforts to provide better information to help patients choose between them, the latest idea being to expand the NHS Choices website to enable patients in England to comment on their GP's performance.[13]

Thus, a framework has been put in place in which NHS organisations must act more like businesses to be financially viable and 'win' customers. Admittedly, this is not a typical market. For one thing, the market has been 'designed', and is performance-managed, by the government. Overall resource allocation and funding is controlled by the state and not the consumer; PCTs do not compete for customers like providers do, they receive block funding from the state to

---

innovation under the Commissioning for Quality and Innovation (CQUIN) scheme.

(e) Polyclinics are essentially super-surgeries, which patients can attend without needing to register. They provide general medical services, but also particular services traditionally provided in hospitals such as X-rays, minor surgery and outpatient treatment.

commission care for patients who live in the geographic area they are responsible for. Second, many characteristics of effective markets are absent.[14] As John Kay explains in his book *The Truth about Markets*, markets work best where the environment is competitive; the consumer has good knowledge of available alternatives and can sensibly make comparative decisions; there is no major information asymmetry either in favour of the consumer or the supplier; the product being bought is a private good, not a public issue; and businesses are free to define their unique selling points, 'select' their customers and, ultimately, go bust if they fail.[15] The NHS 'market' does not fit any of these conditions in any meaningful sense, and some not even partly, so businesses will be facing very different incentives to those in a 'free' market.[(f)]

That said, there is no such thing as a 'stereotypical' market, and the intention behind the current structure is clear. Government reforms to the NHS in England have unquestionably sought to increase the choices available to patients and to stimulate competition between healthcare providers. Frontline organisations that bear the NHS name — particularly foundation trusts — are as much busineses as they are arms of the state. It is only fair, then, to assess how effective such moves have been — and how well our fledgling businesses are doing.

(f) While the public are prepared to accept a branch of Woolworths closing on their high street, they are far less willing to see the local district general hospital (DGH) suffer a similar fate, regardless of the quality of care it offers — which they are unlikely to be privy to in any case.

Commandment One:
Quit Taking Risks

The one outcome that is never measured in the NHS is the outcome of what politicians do.

Polly Toynbee

The NHS was the first universal healthcare system in the world to be free-at-the-point-of-need and has, across its lifetime, contributed to significant improvements in health. In the first 50 years of the NHS, for example, infant mortality fell by more than 80 per cent, the proportion of people dying before the age of 65 fell from 40 per cent to seven per cent and life expectancy rose by a decade.[1]

However, it is commonly acknowledged that despite such achievements the NHS lags behind health systems in other developed countries in the adoption and diffusion of new technologies, innovation and working practices; and is inferior in many areas.[2] Consider a few examples: the NHS fits only 430 new pacemakers per million of the population compared with 900 per million in France, Germany, Belgium and Spain,[3] despite cardiac arrhythmia being one of the top ten causes of unplanned hospital admissions in the UK.[4] Over 40,000 patients in Germany use insulin pumps rather than self-administered injections to manage diabetes, compared with less than 2,000 in the UK.[5] And, as of 2007, the UK had just 4.1 units of radiotherapy equipment per million of the population, which provided some 63 per cent fractions per million of the population less than required according to the government's cancer tsar.[6] The OECD average is 6.2 units per million.[7] In total, the Medical Technology Group estimates that the UK spends just 0.36 per cent of its GDP (and 4.8 per cent of all healthcare expenditure) on medical technology, compared with the European average of 0.55 per cent (6.4 per cent).[8]

11

Figure 1

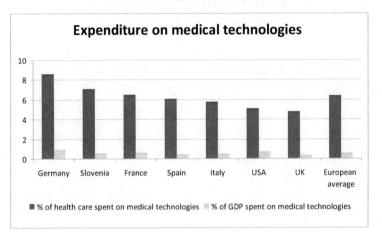

Source: Medical Technology Group (2005)

Some of this, of course, has to do with the historic underfunding of the NHS *vis-à-vis* other health systems. What's more, a certain degree of inertia in some areas where new technology and drugs are concerned may not be a bad thing because many are high-end and—particularly in the case of high-cost drugs—may offer only marginal benefit to patients.[9] Even for technology such as telemedicine, hailed as offering revolutionary potential to transform health care, cost-effectiveness over standard practice is unclear.[10] However, this does not excuse the situation. Where the NHS fails most noticeably is not necessarily in the uptake of *new* technology and drugs, but in the diffusion of those now recognised as clinically effective; and in the adoption of, and willingness to try, new systems and ways of working. At the local level, NHS organisations tend to be profoundly risk-averse.

There are many reasons for this. Health care—with an insurance function, heavy regulation, powerful professional interests and its sheer complexity—is frequently criticised on

12

a global scale for being overly conservative.[11] In many respects this is understandable: introducing new procedures in health care without due care and diligence will not just lose you customers, but kill and disable. However, the literature is fairly clear that the propensity to avoid innovation and risk is not just a function of the industry we happen to be looking at (the catastrophic consequences for failure are the same in the airline industry, for example, yet this has been a highly innovative sphere), but is also determined by things such as a productive organisational structure, capacity and politics; competition; social networks; leadership; communication; and how well organisations actually assess risks.[12]

It is here that the NHS comes up short. At the coal face, organisational culture tends to be isolated, defensive and unconducive to quality improvement. Andrew Mawson's experience in setting up the Bromley-by-Bow Centre, a revolutionary health centre aimed at tackling numerous community health problems, is a case in point.[13] Built and owned by the people it serves, the vision was to create a truly integrated care system in Bromley-by-Bow (a deprived and under-served area in East London) whose team would include not only health professionals, social workers, education experts, project staff and volunteers, but also artists and musicians. Doctors would be able to offer patients more than just drugs—they would also be able to prescribe around 100 different activities a week and give some the opportunity to set up their own businesses. Lord Mawson wrote in his book about the Centre's struggle to get local NHS organisations on board: 'We may as well have proposed a nuclear weapons facility for the area, given the response we [initially] had'.[14]

Further examples are not difficult to find. In Calderdale, the local medical committee and PCT took four years to create a detailed proposal for phlebotomy services to be provided in GP surgeries rather than solely in hospitals, despite the obvious benefit to patients in terms of distance, time and car parking charges. The total cost of the scheme? Between £100,000 and £200,000 per year out of the PCT's annual budget of around £230 million. In Greater Manchester meticulous plans for new neurological rehabilitation units—that had the backing of hospital managers, clinicians and patients—took a similar amount of time to be approved due to health authorities squabbling over who should bear the costs.[15] Perhaps unsurprisingly, a 2006 study of change capability in the NHS by the Office of Government Commerce gave the NHS a score of just two out of five points for seven of the nine categories assessed.[16]

The million-dollar question is why. Here, we must turn to one of the many paradoxes at the heart of the NHS, for to say the organisation *as a whole* never changes and never takes risks would be wrong. At the national level, the actions of government have ensured that the structure of the NHS has changed at an unenviably fast rate and in a somewhat schizophrenic fashion; the consequences of which go a long way to explain the risk- and change-*aversion* of its many parts. A quick run-through of some of the major initiatives since 2000 reveals this clearly: the separation of function in PCTs; the merging of PCTs; the merging of NHS trusts; the creation of foundation trusts; Connecting for Health (and the National Programme for IT, NPfIT); payment-by-results; patient choice; Choose and Book; practice-based commissioning; improving health and well-being; and the 'world class commissioning' agenda. The ultimate irony is that such systemic reform has largely produced circular progress, reversing the alterations New Labour initially made when they came into power in 1997 and taking the NHS back very close to what the Conservatives left.[17] The purchaser/ provider split was abolished, only to be recreated in a more vigorous form; local health authorities became primary care groups and then primary care trusts as the 'third way' reverted back to the market; and GP fundholding was abandoned only to be revived in the form of practice-based commissioning. While all this has been going on, targets—which organisations miss at their peril—have been set on everything from smoking to waiting times (see commandment five).

Figure 2

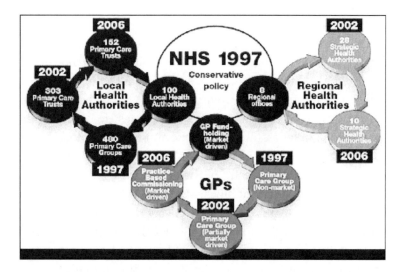

Source: Halligan, L, (2007)

Rotherham PCT's boss, Andy Buck, sums up the resulting situation well: 'we are encouraged to focus on this year—get the finance right, deliver the targets and don't drop any clangers'.[18] Lines of accountability run upwards to the government, rather than downwards to the patient. Instead of being judged by the quality of care they provide for patients, businesses in the NHS are judged by whether they meet central performance targets and can cope with endless restructuring.[19] Too often, they are expected to roll wherever the government chooses to kick them next in order to 'solve' the perceived problem of the moment.

The opportunity cost in terms of the propensity of businesses to innovate and take a few risks has been significant; to cite just one example, academics at King's College London found the merging of NHS trusts typically put performance back by over 18 months.[a] The government are, somewhat paradoxically, aware of this (or at least they see the consequences, without necessarily making the causal connection). At the beginning of 2008, Andy Burnham MP, a former health minister, made an impassioned plea for local organisations to become risk-takers: 'innovate and break traditional patterns of local spending where necessary', he said. 'Common sense is always needed. Don't wait forever for an "evidence base". Change sometimes doesn't happen because people assume innovation might be blocked by central government, but that won't be the case.'[20] However, this is a misunderstanding of the situation. It is not so much that central government blocks attempts to innovate (though it does, and has), but that hyperactivity on the part of central government tends to produce local acquiescence and uncertainty and makes proper evaluation of risk incredibly difficult.[b] Even foundation trusts, which one might expect

---

(a) The Audit Commission also recently uncovered a correlation between the performance of PCTs and whether or not they had been reconfigured in the past few years.

(b) At the same time as Andy Burnham was blogging on *Comment is Free*, the government was in the middle of yet another far-reaching

to be an exception with their semi-autonomous status—much more akin to what most economists would term a business—continue to sit on burgeoning aggregate cash balances of as much as £2.3 billion.[21]

The long-term consequences of this are likely to be significant. The act of innovating, of taking risk, of what Trisha Greenhalgh and colleagues have termed inducing 'a novel set of behaviours, routines and ways of working', does not occur at the flick of a switch.[22] Being 'novel', innovating and making change stick require a culture of openness and constant improvement.[23(c)] Minus this, the ideas of so many clinicians and managers will be stymied either for fear of rocking the boat or because windows of opportunity are simply not seen (see commandment nine). Under pressure from constant structural change, it is this culture of openness that few businesses emerging in the 'brave new world' of the NHS have paid adequate attention to. In too many, the risks associated with the development of new services and ways of working are used as an excuse for maintaining the status quo rather than something to be understood and managed. There is—and this is a theme that reoccurs throughout this book—a tragic sense in which people are stifled by the organisations they work in; and that organisations are stifled by the system they are operating in.[24]

---

review of the NHS led by Lord Darzi, which, according to the *British Medical Journal*, paralysed the DH.

(c) It is no accident that innovative companies, such as Apple and Google, tend to be the ones that people admire and want to work for, where job satisfaction is high and staff turnover low.

Commandment Two: Be Inflexible

For this is the tragedy of man — circumstances change, but he doesn't.

Despite Nye Bevan's famous declaration that 'a bed pan dropped in Tredegar Miners' Hospital will echo down the corridors of Whitehall', the NHS was founded on the principle (or 'concordat') that the government would fund health care but leave its operational running to frontline organisations and staff.[1] In a speech given a few weeks after he became Minister of Health, Bevan said:

> I conceive it the function of the Ministry of Health to provide the medical profession with the best and most modern apparatus of medicine and to enable them to freely use it, in accordance with their training, for the benefit of the people of their country. Every doctor must be free to use that apparatus without interference from secular organisations.[2]

As governments and secretaries of state have come and gone, this ideal has been progressively eroded. A part of this is no doubt understandable. We live in an audit society, where demands for data and accountability are very different from those in 1948; and the dawn of evidence-based medicine has produced calls for government and regulatory bodies to intervene in order to address unacceptable variations in practice. At times, the medical profession has also been guilty of preferring the status quo for no other reason than self-interest. The image of the consultant working in the private sector on NHS time is a powerful one — if mainly a caricature.

However, while all governments have surely had worthy aims for the NHS, the net effect of their desire to exact change and drive performance has led to a situation in which, in 2005, the then Secretary of State for Health, Patricia

Hewitt MP, conceded 'the NHS is four times the size of the Cuban economy and more centralised'.[3] A look at the level of state control over the factors of production used by fledgling businesses in the NHS shows how it tends, perhaps unsurprisingly, to be just as bureaucratic and inflexible.

Staff pay and contracts

Every year, physician and staff pay is negotiated and set centrally based on the recommendations of three national bodies, the NHS Pay Review Body (for all NHS staff employed under Agenda for Change contracts), the Review Body on Doctors' and Dentists' Remuneration and the Senior Salaries Review Body (for very senior managers). Although foundation trusts are able to offer performance pay incentives and Agenda for Change offers a degree of flexibility to all bodies, NHS organisations must ultimately stay within the national pay scales set by the government. This produces numerous problems where pay bands do not fit well with local labour markets. Although the bands vary from region to region, they are not sufficiently adjusted. For example, wages are just 11 per cent higher in the NHS in Inner London than in low-cost areas of the country, compared with an outside wage differential of closer to 60 per cent; a fact that has perverse consequences for quality of care. Academic studies have shown that a ten per cent increase in the outside wage is associated with a four to eight per cent increase in death rates from acute myocardial infarction (AMI). This has been attributed to an increased reliance on temporary agency staff, as NHS trusts in high-wage areas have been unable to increase (regulated) wages to attract permanent employees.[4]

On top of this the contracts within which staff pay is constrained are—with a few exceptions such as the APMS and PMS contracts for GPs—also negotiated centrally, this time by the DH. While guaranteeing a degree of consistency and lowering local bargaining costs, this has nonetheless made it more difficult for local organisations to offer incentives to attract doctors into deprived areas (helping to entrench the Inverse Care Law[a]).[5] It also tends to lock consultants into their hospitals and GPs into their surgeries, when new integrated models of care—particularly the proposed Integrated Care Organisations[b]—demand more flexible ways of working.[6]

To complete the picture, regulation of the medical and nursing profession is increasingly being nationalised. The most poignant example of this is the oversight of the formerly independent General Medical Council (GMC) and Nursing and Midwifery Council (NMC) by a government quango, the Council for Healthcare Regulatory Excellence (CHRE); and the increased role of government in the training of junior doctors. The latter, in particular, has revealed the limits of central control. Modernising Medical

---

(a) The Inverse Care Law was first articulated in 1971 in the medical journal *The Lancet* by Dr Julian Tudor Hart. It states that that 'the availability of good medical care tends to vary inversely with the need for it in the population served'.

(b) ICOs form part of the recommendations of Lord Darzi's *Next Stage Review* of the NHS (2008) and are seen as a means of achieving improved co-ordination of care, delivering better services between secondary, primary and social care, and providing improved overall care for patients more economically. The methods used are likely to vary widely, according to the makeup and needs of local health economies. They include partnerships, new systems and care pathways that span primary, community, secondary and social care.

Careers (MMC) had a worthy aim: to reform postgraduate medical education and training to speed up the production of competent specialists. But wrapped in unclear policy objectives, hampered by a lack of clarity around doctors' roles and conducted through another quango, the Postgraduate Medical and Education Training Board (PMETB), it was—not to put too fine a point on it—a disaster. Represented in the public mind by the fiasco over the application system, MTAS, the whole episode left thousands of junior doctors without posts and was described by the Royal College of Physicians as 'the worst episode in the history of medical training in the UK in living memory'.[7(c)]

Capital

Capital expenditure, with the exception of that by foundation trusts, is tightly constrained by the DH and, in turn, HM Treasury, which sets delegated limits to capital investment across the NHS. Capital plans developed by PCTs and NHS trusts must be agreed with their SHAs, and then by the DH in order to fall within the Department's capital spending limit (for 2009/09 there is £500 million pot to fund local PCT capital schemes).[8] Once agreed, PCTs and NHS trusts are then under a statutory duty to meet their defined capital resource thresholds.

Local freedom over capital expenditure is also curtailed by the requirement of PCTs and NHS trusts to support

---

(c) In 2008 the recruitment process was handed from MMC back to the 13 deaneries, which subsequently adopted a series of smaller online application systems. As of February 2009, over 18,000 applications had been successfully completed.

capital investment decisions made outside their boards (usually by the government or DH), that may or may not be useful. The archetype of this is National Programme for IT (NPfIT), which, as a central programme, has created something of a monopoly on IT that has often crowded out more appropriate local solutions. Seven years ago, for example, Southend Hospital piloted a system that helped ensure drugs were administered to the right patient at the right time, in the right quantity, while also providing doctors with immediate information (and warnings) on possible contra-indications associated with the prescription of multiple drugs. It received a glowing independent review from the Royal Pharmaceutical Society of Great Britain. Despite pleas from doctors, nurses and pharmacists, the government insisted NPfIT would have the answers and the project was abandoned.[9]

It is now unclear that NPfIT will ever deliver on its promise. Already, the project is over-budget and at least four years behind, with expenditure predicted to reach a minimum of £12.4 billion by 2013/14.[10] In the opinion of one IT expert, 'the fundamental dilemma facing NPfIT is that one can (with difficulty) achieve any two of (a) high security, (b) sophisticated functionality, and (c) great scale—but achieving all three is currently, and may well remain, beyond the state of the art'.[11] David Nicholson, the NHS Chief Executive, recently conceded as much in evidence to the House of Commons Health Committee: 'if we don't make progress relatively soon', he said, 'we are really going to have to think it through again'.[(d)12]

(d) Just recently, Andrew Way, the former chief executive of the Royal Free Hospital, that piloted the electronic patient record in London, said the installation had cost the trust £10 million and affected patient services.

The crux of the issue is that effectiveness of IT, as with all capital expenditure, depends not just on 'techie' issues, but on people having confidence in the new technology/ buildings/facilities and being able to use them properly. This requires the engagement of healthcare professionals and a sense of ownership, which is best achieved by there being the flexibility for things to grow from the bottom up. In spite of NPfIT, for example, Heart of England NHS Foundation Trust, through allowing locally talented IT technicians to work with various clinical enthusiasts and 'splice together their unique systems with the best of what is out there', is already reaching the point where some specialties can manage without paper records.[13] Why not extend the freedom to retain annual surpluses and invest without delegated limits to all organisations?[(e)]

Rationing

Wherever collective responsibility is taken for health care there will inevitably be rationing of services for the simple economic reason that budgets are finite. However, because the NHS is a single-payer system that does not permit top-up payments for the most marginal treatments, there has been pressure to centralise this function, hence the birth of the National Institute for Health and Clinical Excellence

---

(e) Unfortunately, the recent financial turmoil has made it only too clear where the buck stops. It has HM Treasury greedily eyeing the surpluses that allow foundation trusts to pursue such schemes; the November Pre-Budget Report 'identified' £100 million per annum that could be saved in the NHS by improving the use of the estate; and the DH apparently intends to pressure PCTs to sell their property in order to fill a £5 billion black hole in its capital spending limit.

(NICE). To be fair, this has brought many benefits. The importance of evidence-based medicine and the realities of finite resources have been brought into the open, and NICE has provided something of a solution to the 'no-win' situation the government finds itself in when it comes to 'postcode prescribing'.[f]

However, NICE has also created real difficulties for local organisations, predominantly because it makes its recommendations in isolation from PCT budgets and at some distance from day-to-day decision-making. In particular, NICE makes few allowances for the fact that any guidance it issues mandating NHS organisations to prescribe X drug or Y treatment will come at an opportunity cost for local programmes.[14] These may have to be withdrawn and, by proxy, an organisation's ability to be flexible in response to local need is restricted. The implications of this are put starkly by Sophia Christie, Chief Executive of Birmingham East and North PCT:

> We are currently planning to invest £12m in a range of large service developments which have been through a rigorous process of needs assessment, targeting, piloting and testing before comprehensive roll-out. If we spend £4m on Lucentis [following NICE guidance] it will be at the expense of the redesign and expansion of end of life care; significant investment in rehabilitation in partnership with the local authority; and making assertive telephone management available to 11,000 more people struggling with long-term conditions.[15]

Yet, if the PCT doesn't conform to the guidance they will be accused of preventing access to treatment. This is not an easy choice to make.

(f) Postcode prescribing refers to a situation where a PCT in one part of the country agrees to pay for a particular job, but others do not.

The net result of such state control over factors of production is too often organisational paralysis and silo-working (see commandment three). When control over factors of production is centralised in the hands of a few at the top of the chain, rather than in the many businesses that make it up, the temptation to use it is immense; and so it has proved in the NHS. Lip-service is paid to local decision-making, but in reality this is only allowed if central requirements have been met and the relevant forms have been filled in (see commandments five and eight). The Nuffield Trust think-tank recently outlined eight major functions of quality reform in the NHS over the past ten years, from standard-setting and monitoring to public reporting, and provided at least 24 examples of discrete reforms within this.[16] The proposals in Lord Darzi's *Next Stage Review* of the NHS, published in 2008, will only add to this. At least 40 major changes are floated—from new services to new directorships, frameworks and standards— all under the false promise of no new targets or organi-sational change.[17]

In any public health system there will inevitably be a role for government in setting priorities and disseminating guidance—creating National Service Frameworks (NSFs) to focus attention on key disease areas such as coronary heart disease, has, for example, yielded results—but the freedom for local organisations and teams of clinicians to deliver must forever remain. Without it, a dependency culture is fostered that is hard to shift and the flexibility to respond to the different needs of patients is lost. So—as we shall see throughout this book—it has been in the NHS.[18]

Commandment Three:
Isolate Yourself

Interfaces of care are dangerous places for patients.

Mayur Lakhani and Maureen Baker

It is often assumed that the NHS, being a single-payer health system, is the ultimate integrated healthcare organisation. However, one of the most frequent complaints of patients is of being 'lost in the system'. The search for seamless care, as the Performance Director of the DH Richard Gleave put it, remains something of a holy grail.[1]

As ever, there are multiple reasons for this. Akin to all health systems, the NHS suffers the consequences of battles between powerful professional interests; between the conflicting priorities of clinicians and managers;[a][2] and between provider and purchaser organisations—most frequently over the allocation of resources, or the use of evidence-based medicine and quality improvement strategies. With responsibility for funding, provision and resource allocation ultimately lying with the government, NHS businesses also operate in a uniquely political environment. The DH is often guilty of accusing doctors of being (and assuming that they are) 'vested producer interests' whenever plans do not work; and doctors are unashamed of launching virulent attacks on government policy.[b]

(a) The root of this conflict is different priorities: managers are predominantly focused on population groups, efficiency and the government agenda, and clinicians on treating individual patients.

(b) To give a flavour of this often juicy but largely unproductive dispute, in 2007 the British Medical Association (BMA) went so far

However, the biggest source of isolation and subsequent breakdown in the continuity of patient care is the artificial divide between primary and secondary care.[c] The division is largely historical and has existed since (and before) the NHS was founded, but there is a sound case to be made that recent reforms have made it worse. As Jennifer Dixon and Sir Cyril Chantler have put it:

> The incentives in the system are not appropriate, being mainly designed to reduce waiting lists (i.e. to increase volumes of surgical cases moving through hospitals), not to reduce avoidable admissions—for example, through better management of medical conditions in primary care. Hospitals are paid a fixed national price for an admission based on diagnosis and are encouraged to admit more patients and to expand services that create a surplus rather than necessarily meet need or deliver the most cost-effective outcomes... The levers for PCTs to manage demand for hospital care are weak, and support of, and engagement by, [GPs involved in] practice-based commissioning is low... hospital specialists do not receive financial encouragement to work with general

---

as to accuse the government of 'a woeful dereliction of duty towards patients, towards the profession and towards the future' (in a press release); and Alan Johnson, the Secretary of State for Health chose to release the NHS Constitution on the premise of 'ending the era of doctor knows best'. When Health Minister Ben Bradshaw recently proclaimed (8 March 2009) to the *Sunday Telegraph* that GPs 'could be forced out of the NHS if they do not adhere to rules which say they should offer their patients a choice of where to go for hospital care', the leader of the BMA, Dr Hamish Meldrum, responded by accusing the government of 'bullyboy tactics and megaphone diplomacy'.

(c) A similar point could be made of the division between health care, which is the responsibility of the NHS, and social care, which is the responsibility of local government. However, for sake of space and experience if nothing else, we have decided to focus on that between primary and secondary care.

practitioners and others, and consequently care is often not integrated.[3]

The crux of the issue is that the incentives facing primary and secondary care organisations are more at odds with each other than aligned, which, when it comes to optimum care for patients, does not make for a happy place. The problems experienced by patients when moving from one stage of care to another across interfaces or between professionals are numerous and well documented, astutely described by one set of academics as 'getting in', 'fitting in', 'knowing what's going on', 'continuity' and 'limbo'.[4] Patients must gain access to care (obtaining appointments, being referred, going through admission procedures in hospital and receiving after-care). This must then be consistent, coordinated and appropriate to their needs. And patients must receive understandable and accurate information about the care they are receiving. Too often, however, the experience of patients is of being left 'in limbo'. Organisational barriers to relational continuity (such as being able to book an appointment to see your GP) and managerial continuity (such as the coordination of care across primary and secondary care) are significant; and communication, both between sites of care and between those sites and patients, is poor.[5] For patients with a number of complaints—particularly those with multiple chronic conditions who must access a greater number of points of care—such barriers can get unmanageable. The experience of this patient, with chronic obstructive pulmonary disease (COPD) and renal failure, is not atypical:

> P: ... they are still getting no results... [the consultant] wanted to prescribe me these two types of tablets for the heart problem... But because of the renal problems that I had he couldn't prescribe me one of the tablets until he got the results of the blood tests. So he phoned up my GP surgery for the blood tests, they didn't have it...

Anyway, I had to wait then, they done [sic] blood tests on me at [the hospital] that day but he had to wait then a week to get the results of the blood tests back and then contact my GP for him to prescribe me the other type of tablets he wanted me on... and I was up then [at] the end of January for the renal clinic again and they hadn't got it again.[6]

A particular bone of contention is informational discontinuity following hospital discharge. According to surveys by the NHS Alliance (a primary care group) over the past three years, 70 per cent of GP practices experience late discharge summaries 'very often' or 'fairly often';[(d)] delays which 90 per cent of GPs said compromised clinical care and 68 per cent said compromised patient safety.[7] A similar statistic would be true for miscommunication between healthcare organisations *per se*.[8]

However, such isolation is not just a question of patient safety; it is also one of quality and cost. One of the biggest cost drivers in the NHS is emergency hospital admissions for chronic conditions (such as asthma) and acute conditions (such as ear, nose and throat infections) that are usually — and typically optimally — managed in primary care. Both have increased over the past five years in England, the rate for acute conditions quite dramatically so from 371.57

(d) To take two examples, in Halifax last year the medical unit did a catch up on discharge summaries, after which one of the authors (PD) received a communication in November 2008 about significant acute medical events that happened five months earlier. Earlier in the year, several sacks of clinical mail — with details of patients, their results, their operations, their medical conditions and their follow up appointments — were lost in the post room cupboard in Leeds General Infirmary, yet GPs did not start to wonder why they had not heard anything until 4-8 weeks later.

admissions per 100,000 persons in 2002/03 to 423.40 in 2006/07.[9]

Figure 3

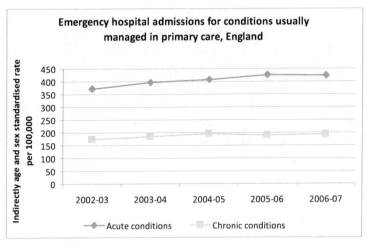

Source: NCHOD (2008)

While the reasons for this are unclear, it does suggest that the disjuncture between primary and secondary care is—at the very least—not improving, which is likely to have knock-on effects on quality. There is increasing recognition that greater integration—defined by the World Health Organisation (WHO) as 'bringing together inputs, delivery, management and organisation of services relating to diagnosis, treatment, care, rehabilitation and health promotion'[10] —breeds excellence. Evidence suggests patients garner greater benefit, and are more satisfied, when referrals are co-ordinated and managed well.[11] Within the NHS, research by Sheffield University has identified the benefits of urgent care networks; and examples such as Bolton PCT's managed diabetes network, Epsom Downs Integrated Care Services (EDICS) and the Central Middlesex Hospital's approach (see below) show the advantages of the integrated management of people with chronic disease across primary/secondary care.[12] The most comprehensive evidence, however, comes from the USA. Large integrated health organisations—such as Kaiser Permanente, the Veterans Health Administration (VHA) and the Mayo Clinic—and other more medium-sized organisations—such as Geisinger in Pennsylvania and Health Partners in Minnesota—are gaining significant international attention.[13] Through integrating governance, risk management, frontline services and information technology, such organisations have been able to develop a single culture spanning primary, secondary and community services that is dedicated to high quality, cost-effective care.[14] Despite controversies over the comparability of data, it is increasingly acknowledged that the outcomes they achieve—clinical, patient-centred and efficiency related—are superior to the NHS. Though vigorously disputed in some quarters, one study estimated that age-adjusted rates of acute hospital service use in Kaiser Permanente were one third less than in the NHS.[15]

The most important characteristic of such integrated healthcare organisations, however, is their ability to see things from the patient's perspective and develop services accordingly. A patient's experience of health care is continuous, it does not stop and start every time they cross between interfaces of care or see a different physician. Some NHS organisations are attempting to change to such a philosophy. The Healthcare Commission recently complimented a number of PCTs that had well-established networks of community groups—particularly for those with specific diseases such as diabetes and cancer—to feed people's views into commissioning boards. The Royal College of Physicians and the Royal College of General Practitioners also uncovered over 300 instances of new models of working in the community involving specialists and generalists, from respiratory medicine to co-located urgent care for children.[16] And there are cases, such as the Central Middlesex Hospital's attempts to merge primary and secondary care for patients with chronic diseases, which serve as a pointer to more comprehensive solutions.[17]

Yet these are exceptions rather than the rule. Few businesses in the NHS routinely take account of people's views when planning and improving services, and one of the most common complaints of patients is the difficulty of trying to make their views heard.[18] Even where patient views are sought and clear aims are expressed, the barriers to change are significant. Central Middlesex, for example, found it very difficult to break down organisational, cultural and professional barriers to integrating primary and secondary services, not least dealing with income loss from reducing avoidable admissions.[19] Either for reasons of 'comfort' or misplaced initiatives, it is far easier for NHS businesses to isolate themselves and continue to work in their respective silos. High quality health care may be provided in one 'part' of the chain, but disjoints between them are likely to result in mistakes when the pathway is taken as a whole. As one patient said, 'you feel a bit like an accessory... you've got this great big medical system and you're really not part of it, the system rolls on whether you're there or not'.[20]

Commandment Four:
Assume Infallibility

What should they know of England, who only England know?

Rudyard Kipling

When researching his history of The King's Fund, the distinguished historian Frank Prochaska discovered that in the 1930s British voluntary hospitals were widely accepted as 'the best in the world'.[1] That phrase, or its variant, 'envy of the world', has lingered on from the pre-NHS era—often regardless of the evidence. Upon its 60th anniversary in 2008, the Prime Minster described the NHS as the 'pride of Britain',[2] and Ann Keen, a health minister, reported to the House of Commons: 'it continues to be the envy of the world'.[3] In a recent ICM poll of the public for the BBC, 51 per cent of respondents apparently agreed with her.[4]

The problem with such claims is that relatively few people—clinicians, managers or patients—in England know much about standards of treatment, access to health care and funding systems used in the rest of the world. When politicians argue in favour of the NHS they often (rightly) draw unfavourable comparisons with the US system, but in doing so give the false impression that this is the only international alternative. Health outcomes are notoriously difficult to measure, and their causes are complex, but when data on UK performance is compared with other models of universal health care across continental Europe, describing the NHS as 'the envy of the world' reveals a good deal about British parochialism.

(i)   Although above-average improvement was registered between 1997/98 and 2002/03, analysis by Ellen Nolte and Martin McKee at the London School of Hygiene and Tropical Medicine puts the UK 16th out of 19

33

industrialised countries in terms of **amenable mortality** (a vital measure of health system performance that tries to remove external influences on health by accounting for deaths from certain causes before age 75 that are potentially preventable with timely and effective health care). One-hundred-and-three deaths per 100,000 of the population were considered preventable in the UK, compared with just 65 in the best performing country, France.[5]

Figure 4

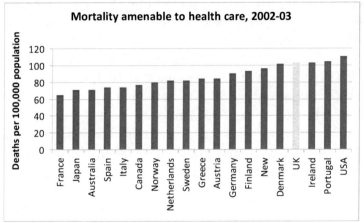

Mortality amenable to health care, 2002-03

Source: Nolte, E, and McKee, M, (2008)

(ii)   The NHS remains at the foot of European league tables in terms of **five-year survival rates from one of the biggest killers, cancer,** much closer to the performance of Poland and the Czech Republic than those with the best outcomes, the Nordic countries.[6] What's more, despite the introduction of the NHS Cancer Plan in 2000, there have been only small improvements in one-year survival for many cancers,[7]

34

while domestic improvements in amenable mortality for cancer actually *fell* year-on-year between 2000/01 and 2004/05.[8]

(iii) A number of international multicentre trials looking at **stroke care** in Western European countries have found the worst outcomes in the UK, even when adjusting for case mix and use of healthcare resources.[9] In one study the difference in the proportion of patients dead or dependent between the UK and the other eight countries was between 150 and 300 events per 1,000 patients.[10]

(iv) **Life expectancy and social equity** are comparatively low and **infant mortality** comparatively high in the UK compared with other developed countries.[11] (Table 1, p. 39.)

(v) According to **surveys of patients** in 30 European countries by the Brussels-based Health Consumer Powerhouse, the NHS is also some way behind the best performers on more patient-focused measures, such as patient rights and information, e-health, waiting time for treatment, the range and reach of services, and access to pharmaceuticals. In 2008 the UK was positioned 13th overall with 650 points, compared with France, the top-scoring country, which achieved a score of 839.[12]

Domestically, surveys by the Picker Institute have shown that while NHS care has improved significantly in some important respects (particularly waiting times), the service as a whole is still far from patient-centred, with the most significant problem being the failure of clinical staff to provide active support for patient engagement.[13]

Inevitably, analysis of the reasons behind these discrepancies is difficult; data comparability, differences in climate and lifestyle, culture, historic health spending and mere accidents of history all come into play.[14] However, some of the difference may well be explained by the fact that few other countries have health systems that are so centralised, monopolistic and subject to politicised management as the NHS.[15] Many of the best performers in Europe—while equally committed to universal provision and social solidarity—do not fund health care through taxation, but through social insurance. In such systems there is a much closer link between health spending and outcomes, because premiums are paid to insurers rather than the government, and patients typically have a far greater choice of provider. As a result, both insurers (the equivalent of PCTs in England) and providers have a strong incentive to value patients—if they don't they will lose custom.[16] Typically, this also affords a greater respect for professional autonomy because it is less compromised by government interference.[17] The idea of a hospital chief executive, despite now in effect running a business, being forced to resign as a result of a hard line towed by government or SHAs on targets is comparatively alien to the social insurance model.[a][b]

(a) In February 2009, for example, two chief executives of London hospital trusts resigned amidst pressure from NHS London on key targets, prompting the chair of UCLH Foundation Trust to declare 'there's a Stalinist culture that isn't helpful'.

(b) For other high-performing systems that do fund health care through taxation, such as Sweden and Denmark, responsibility for provision is typically devolved to local government and councils with central government departments having more of a supervisory role.

In the NHS, however, the situation is very different. The favourite catchphrase of the NHS chief executive David Nicholson is for NHS boards to 'look outwards to their local communities, not upwards to Whitehall', but this is essentially empty rhetoric while the accountability of PCTs and NHS trusts (that aren't foundation trusts) continues to run upward through SHAs to the DH. The prevalent culture is one of 'central credit, local blame'. The centre is happy to take the credit for the NHS's achievements,[18] but when the uptake of patient choice is low, when those in the service are aghast at government plans, or when PCTs are struggling to meet the competencies laid out by the DH, it tends to be the clinician's or manager's fault.[19] As Norman Lamb MP, the Liberal Democrat health spokesperson, has noted: '95 per cent of taxes are raised centrally [in the UK], compared with the EU average of 60 per cent. Power [tends to] reside where money is raised.'[20]

The NHS's aims have always been laudable, and remain so today; a lack of money should never prevent anyone suffering the misfortune of ill health from getting quality treatment. But, we should not assume the infallibility of the current system. In doing so, we risk sleepwalking into a world of misnomers and a false rationale for pursuing endless superficial reform at the cost of change—both systemic and patient-level—that could be truly beneficial. NHS organisations are now expected to act like businesses and focus on tailoring services to patients, but frequently find themselves operating in a system that, when it comes down to it, does not really want them to. Progress has been made over the past ten years, but—as we shall see in the next commandment—it has been achieved largely through bullying, incremental change and increasing capacity, rather than by genuinely embracing new ways of working and focusing on developing cultures that support continuous quality improvement.[21]

Table 1: Healthcare Characteristics of Leading Economies

Country	% GDP spent on health (1=greatest percentage)	WHO ranking	Life expectancy rank (1-highest LE)	Cancer mortality rank (1=lowest mortality)	Infant mortality (1=lowest mortality)	Social equity (1=highest equity towards poor)
Japan	7=	2	1	2	1	1 (predicted)
Switzerland	2	5	2=	1	2=	2
France	3	1	4	6	2=	7
Germany	4	6	5=	5	2=	5
Australia	6	7	2=	3	6=	3
Netherlands	5	3	5=	8	2=	6
UK	7=	4	7	7	6=	8
USA	1	8	8	4	8	4

Source: Bosanquet, N. et al., *Making the NHS the Best Insurance Policy in the World*, London: Reform, 2008.

Commandment Five:
Play Game Close to Foul Line

When a measure becomes a target, it ceases to be a measure.

Goodhart's Law

Despite improvements in technology and new fads in management, all business ultimately boils down to matters of trust—that customers trust the product or service will do what it promises, that investors trust management to be competent and that employees trust management to live up to its obligations.[1] Once any of these links is compromised, so is the business: think Enron, Northern Rock... the entire banking system.

In health care this is even more important. Good medicine is premised on values as much as technical expertise: on kindness, caring, effective clinical knowledge, good communication, honesty, and above all on trust.[2] Clinicians hold trust as currency; their whole existence is predicated on trusting what patients tell them, and on patients trusting what clinicians say and do. Without it, symptoms will be missed, diagnoses not made and treatment plans not followed through; the doctor/patient relationship is nothing, and medical care cannot function. Yet across the NHS that trust is in a parlous state: as the case of Mid Staffordshire NHS Foundation Trust has proved, a hospital can be ticking all the boxes, be rated 'good' on quality of care, yet still utterly fail patients.

One of the underlying causes is that NHS organisations— despite being set up as businesses—have been forced to play the game far too close to the foul line. Endless streams of regulation, targets and standards have been preferred by policymakers as the postmodern alternative to moral probity. At the peak following the publication of the NHS

Plan in 2000, managers reckoned they had to meet 300-plus targets,[3] causing even the former Secretary of State for Health Frank Dobson to remark that 'if everything is to be a priority, nothing will be a priority'.[4] The number of headline targets has subsequently been reduced, but the demands of policy documents, operating frameworks and regulatory bodies have acted as sufficient counter-balance. The Healthcare Commission's Annual Health Check last year alone assessed hospital trusts against 44 standards, 33 existing national targets and 36 new national targets; as well as their use of resources.[5] In primary care, general practice is examined against the 135 indicators relating to clinical and organisational quality that make up the Quality and Outcomes Framework (QOF).[6] This is a dangerous place to be heading. 'Trust', as the philosopher Onora O'Neill has shrewdly observed, 'seems to have receded as transparency has advanced.'[7]

Of course, there is evidence that targets and performance management by the centre have induced change. Biomedical quality on indicators included in the QOF has improved since its introduction;[8] waiting times have fallen for inpatients, outpatients, in A&E, and across the referral-to-treatment (RTT) pathway;[9] increases in staff numbers and facilities have followed targeted trajectories;[10] and rates of MRSA and *C. difficile* are falling.[11] We have never had it so good. However, as the Royal Statistical Society warned in 2004:

> It is usually inept to set an extreme-value target, such as 'no patient shall wait in accident and emergency for more than four hours', because as soon as one patient waits in A&E for more than four hours, the target is foregone and thereafter irrelevant. Typically, avoiding extremes consumes disproportionate resources.[12]

The worst example of this is the 18-week referral-to-treatment target. When it was set, the government admitted

41

neither they, nor anyone else, had any idea how ambitious it was, how attainable it was, nor how much it would cost, because at the time the NHS had never collected the relevant data.[13]

Targets, to adopt Keough's terminology, encourage organisations to play far too close to the foul line. They create a 'must-win' scenario that, focusing on only one part of the process rather than the whole, is unlikely to yield high quality care for the individual patient.[14] Visible data will confirm the target has been met, and will be taken as evidence of good performance, but blind spots are numerous and the true impact is concealed. Anything outside the metric is neither seen nor registered.

In A&E, official statistics show nearly 98 per cent of patients turned around in under the four-hour target,[15] but academics have used queuing theory—a mathematical analysis of waiting time statistics—to show this can only have been achieved by 'the employment of dubious management tactics'.[16] Well documented examples, confirmed in surveys by the British Medical Association (BMA),[17] include moving patients to 'clinical decision units' (the four-hour clock stops, even though proper assessment has not been carried out); making patients wait in ambulances (the four-hour clock only starts when the A&E threshold is crossed); admitting patients unnecessarily; discharging people too early and miscoding data.[18] In electives, after inpatient and outpatient waiting time targets were introduced, median waits increased, waiting time was shifted to diagnostics[19] and bed occupancy rose to levels associated with excessive risk of infection.[20] In general practice, after targets were set for offering patients a GP appointment within 48 hours, up to 30 per cent of patients found they were no longer able to book an appointment more than three days in advance.[21] While the QOF targeted biomedical indicators in the treatment of particular diseases, quality of care for those with complex co-morbidities and conditions not included in the framework has shown comparatively little improvement.[22] Last, but not least, the eight-minute response time target for ambulance crews has been widely criticised for holding back service improvement, such as referring and treating more patients out of hospital.[23]

The most pernicious outcome of all of this has been the ill-effect on the ability of health professionals and businesses to develop a self-improving culture that truly puts patients at centre-stage. In becoming the only thing that matters, what is being measured is actually becoming meaningless.[a] Instead of fostering the ability to learn, pressure to score short-term goals has left measurement associated with spin, selection and punishment.[24] Attention has been focused on hitting targets, rather than the feelings, emotions and actual journey an individual patient experiences.[25] Quality, in essence, is determined against crude indicators, not the expectations and experience of those using the service. While performance measures—as we shall see in the next commandment—have their place, they must be appropriately formulated and both locally and clinically owned. To revisit the example of A&E, why, for example, is no-one asking why patients are there in the first place; whether they are actually on the road to recovery; whether the rapid transfer from A&E has actually just left patients waiting

---

(a) This is the essence of Goodhart's Law: that once a social or economic indicator or other *surrogate* measure is made a target for the purpose of conducting social or economic policy then it will lose the information content that would qualify it to play such a role.

elsewhere (and for longer); and whether their experience has been a good one?[26]

The biggest challenge now facing fledgling businesses in the NHS is cultural change. They must move away from playing close to the foul line and refocus on patients and the values they hold so dear, on renewing trust and on reviving what, in essence, is the first purpose of clinical medicine: to relieve human suffering.[27] This will not be easy and will take time. Years of focusing on central initiatives is not an easy habit to break; practice has either become so ingrained it's difficult to see things differently, or staff acquiesce because they've tried so many times to change the system and got nowhere. But there should be no choice: if the old model of command-and-control has failed, managers and healthcare professionals must grasp what opportunities exist and seek to deliver. As Jack Welch, former CEO of General Electric—possibly the world's most successful corporation—said: 'the people closest to the work know the work best'.

Commandment Six:
Don't Take Time to Think

A man who does not think for himself does not think at all.

Oscar Wilde

The German philosopher Johann von Goethe once said: 'the hardest thing to see is what is in front of your eyes'. Any clinician, manager or chief executive involved in attempting to drive improvement in health care will tell you that no matter how well-hatched a plan is, the hazards and uncertainties lying in wait will be significant, inescapable and can only be tackled with an open mind. Quality is not explained by lists of factors and processes, but by the complex interactions between them; it is not just a question of putting the right structures and processes in place and sitting back and watching improvement unfold.[1] Nor can top-down change led by distant organisations such as the DH ever be truly effective. People work in organisations; and it's impossible to ignore organisational, human and cultural dimensions to change.[2] As the President of the Institute for Healthcare Improvement Donald Berwick has written: 'nothing about effective action is "installable" without constant, recursive adjustments to ever-changing local context'.[3] In the context of the NHS, then, effective change is best led by local businesses, that must embody leadership, but also nous, intelligence, hard work, vision, and above all thought.

At the macro-level, however, the NHS has tended to work against this. The NHS's history has been less of well-coordinated approaches that take into account the complexities of change, more a tale of recurrent problems, trial and error, and hastily cobbled-together solutions.[4] Why, one might ask? At root there are two key problems. First, the politicised and heavily centralised nature of the service. As commandments one and five revealed, the desire to be seen to 'do something' tends to create a penchant for quick-wins that is frequently detrimental to service delivery. But second (and some would say as a consequence of this), because the NHS has never worked to a clear definition of 'health', businesses operating in the NHS have an incoherent idea of what they are supposed to achieve.[5] Is the goal to keep people healthy; to reduce 'health inequalities';[(a)] to help solve societal problems that transgress government policy; or simply to help get people better when they are sick?[(b)]

The substitute for this lack of clarity has been a plethora of incoherent initiatives and policy reviews. Too often the DH and others (including academia and think tanks) bring together papers recommending system reform that are actually many different initiatives lashed together, without adequate consideration as to whether or not the sum of such efforts will make sense. Particularly common errors are to:

(a) This term in particular is bandied about with great show, but rarely is it clear whether the speaker is talking about inequalities in incidence of disease, access to treatment or outcomes from disease. It is also unclear as to whether reducing 'health inequalities' should be a legitimate driver of policy, as it seems to come into conflict with the Hippocratic Oath of doctors that says, *inter alia*, that the 'health of my patient will be my first consideration'.

(b) On this point we would say this. The NHS is an organisation that primarily delivers medical and other remedial services; it is not an organisation that can of itself deliver health either on an individual basis or collectively to the nation, as this is mainly a product of social, economic and political factors. As the epidemiologist Richard Wilkinson has pointed out, any healthcare service stands in relation to its patient population somewhat as a military field hospital does to a battle; it patches up the casualties, but—with a few notable exceptions—alone cannot stop them occurring.

ignore the effects a policy may have on different parts of the system; fail to consider the impact a policy will have on people and organisational culture; announce new initiatives before key details have been developed; and overload policy instruments with too many objectives, for which they were not designed.[6] In January 2008, for example, the Prime Minister Gordon Brown announced screening for early signs of heart disease, stroke and kidney disease without any idea of how the programme could be implemented, or how much it might cost.[7]

The best example of recent times, however, is Lord Darzi's 2008 review of the NHS, *High Quality Care for All*. As ever it offers an enticing vision, but as the respected health policy analyst Donald Light commented:

> Even though every proposed change has some merit, none is critically analysed, and the relations between the changes are not examined. There is no discussion of trade-offs, possible harms, wasted funds, knock-on effects, or assessment as would occur in a careful strategic plan.[8]

This is particularly the case with regard to the quality initiatives that are proposed. NICE is to have an expanded role in setting and approving 'more independent quality standards' (a prime example, alongside its new role in assessing the QOF, of overloading a policy instrument that has been relatively successful), but there is also to be a new National Quality Board, new 'Quality Observatories' in each SHA region and a national requirement for NHS (foundation) trusts to publish 'Quality Accounts'. All the while, local clinical teams are to be encouraged 'to develop a wider range of useful local metrics'. It is hard to see how these initiatives and organisations will avoid stepping on each other's toes (particularly given the stake the new Care Quality Commission also has in the field—see commandment eight). There is—as the House of Commons Health

Committee emphasised—no proposed method for evaluating the effectiveness, or cost, of the proposals.[9]

The dangers of such an approach to policymaking are clear: while external influences on quality of care can be overstated, a lack of analysis at the top will inevitably filter down to confusion in frontline business. Everyone in NHS organisations is 'busy' but few have time to stop, think and ask if they are busy doing the right things—if anyone is sure what the right things are. With each new policy initiative requiring more resources to be diverted away from frontline patient care, data production is fast becoming an end in itself rather than a means to drive performance (see commandment eight). Academic research has shown, for example, how wired and controlling central policy has decreased the ability of senior managers to display leadership, to think and to positively affect the delivery of services;[10] and has left governance at board level uncertain, without the focus, skills and cohesion to deliver.[11] Although improvement is being registered, in the latest assessment of use of resources by the Audit Commission, just five per cent of NHS organisations (excluding foundation trusts) were found to be performing strongly (the highest level), with seven per cent failing to meet minimum standards.[12]

Ironically, policymaking and quality improvement strategy could learn a lot from the rigours of the day-to-day practice of medicine. Here, the notion 'I know it will work' or 'my patient knows it works' does not suffice; the drive must always be towards an evidence-base that stands the tests of science (akin to the 'science' or discipline of quality improvement, if you like). Yet at the same time there must always be flexibility: every patient will present with slightly different symptoms, which means effective interpersonal communication, a doctor's experience and his or her ability to apply sound research findings to each patient is vital (the cultural and emotional side of quality improvement in our metaphor).

In other words, policymaking and quality improvement should have an evidence-base and leave ample space for people and organisations to develop knowledge. The source of innovation institutionalised by the Cochrane Collaboration, for example, is not just a powerful critique of complacent and uncritical forms of diagnosis and treatment, but also the delivery and organisation of health care.[13] If you do not measure progress, how will you know that change has brought about improvement and, if there has been improvement, what caused it? As a recent paper by the NHS Confederation argued, 'the power of managerial or system innovation to improve or hold back health care is very considerable'. Terry Young, a professor at Brunel University, goes so far as to say that the use of industrial techniques (such as lean, Plan-Do-Study-Act cycle, statistical process control, six sigma, theory of constraints and mass customisation) and predictive modelling could alone deliver 50-100 per cent more on the same NHS budget.[14]

This is not unrealistic. The use of lean,[(c)15] for example, helped Flinders Medical Centre in Australia do 15 to 20 per cent more work after two-and-a-half years, with fewer safety

---

(c) 'Systems' or 'lean' thinking was pioneered by Taiichi Ohno and saw Toyota become the world-leader in manufacturing. As well as being premised on value to the customer and local leadership lean entails a large amount of attention paid to discussion, analysis and careful testing. Its business culture is one devoted to identifying problems, thinking them through and tackling them before proceeding further. It allows local leaders to evaluate what needs to be done and, at its heart, aims to improve flow and eliminate waste *across* a system by getting the right things to the right place, at the right time, in the right quantities.

incidents, on the same budget, using the same infrastructure, staff and technology. More recently, the same strategy helped Bolton NHS Trust, using less space and fewer resources, to reduce its average turnaround time in pathology from over 24 hours to between two and three.[16] The recent clinical trial involving the use of a short checklist before surgery that—despite the initial scepticism of as many as 50 per cent of the surgeons taking part—led to a remarkable fall in death rates (from 1.5 per cent before its introduction to 0.8 per cent after) and complications (11.0 per cent to 7.0 per cent) was built on pit-stop technology and airline safety initiatives.[17] And, most comprehensively, 'extending the principles of evidence-based medicine to the administrative arena', considering value in terms of the relationship between inputs and outputs, and emphasising clinical leadership, helped transform the Veterans Health Administration (VHA) in the USA over a ten-year period from a low- to high-performing system. Significantly improved outcomes were registered across value domains, with costs simultaneously reduced by more than 25 per cent.[18]

Of course, due care and attention should forever be taken in applying such strategies to health care. Each patient presenting may well be unique, needs are sometimes hard to identify and it is not always clear that one approach is better than another.[19] How quality improvement is implemented is just—if not more important—than the strategy itself: there are many paths up the mountain even if some may be more trodden than others.[20] The cases cited above are just a few examples of what can be achieved given the right environment. What is vital, however, is to recognise the importance that all attached to evidence, thinking and local initiative. The current hyperactive approach of government to health care does little to support this. 'How' as the brilliantly named David Mechanic put it, 'should hamsters run?'[21]

Commandment Seven:
Put Faith in Consultants

Ninety per cent of consultants give the other ten per cent a bad reputation.

Henry A. Kissinger

In 1926 James Oscar McKinsey, a professor at the University of Chicago, set up one of the first management consultancies, McKinsey & Co., which now stands as one of the biggest and most successful in the world. In doing so, he pioneered a more holistic approach to business, incorporating financial fundamentals but also production and marketing. In 1935, however, McKinsey was persuaded to leave his fledgling business to become chief executive of Marshall Field & Co., a large US company. Two years later he tragically died but, reflecting on his experiences on his deathbed, he admitted one thing in particular: that consulting was *much* easier than actually delivering.[1]

This encapsulates the difficulty in using management consultants, especially when it comes to health care with its powerful mix of science and judgement. Many will have considerable expertise in their field—particularly in the various aspects of quality improvement referred to in commandment six—and may have a lot to offer. To cite a concrete example, ten clients of the healthcare intelligence provider CHKS moved from 'fair' to 'excellent' in the Healthcare Commission's Annual Health Check for 2008; with one moving from 'weak' to 'excellent'.[2] However, management consultants in general are unlikely to be around organisations for long and, crucially, are unlikely to be the ones actually leading change in organisations. The problem here is that while management consultants may be useful in providing impulses for change (and offering

51

guidance along the way), high quality health care cannot be bought off the shelf; ultimately it can only be driven by 'players' *within* an organisation. Successful, and sustained, improvement depends less on external stimuli and more on developing an internal culture of learning and service.[3]

For a number of years, however, businesses in the NHS (admittedly often at the behest of the DH, or to conform to central requirements) have often preferred to employ management consultants to gather and analyse information, and to posit reforms and change, rather than do what Keough termed 'watching the bull' themselves. No-one quite knows how much the NHS as a whole spends on management consultants because the information is not collected centrally. However, estimates in 2006 ranged from £325 million[4] to over one per cent of the NHS's budget at £1 billion (the latter was not disputed by the DH).[5] *Accountancy Age* magazine now lists the NHS as the fourth biggest consultancy market in the UK;[6] and, with new opportunities arising through Lord Darzi's review of the NHS and the Framework for Procuring External Support for Commissioners (FESC), it is also something of a growth industry. Yet to our knowledge no large-scale analysis has been carried out on value for money. Problems in major projects such as NPfIT (see commandment two) could have provided the impetus to do so, but did not,[7] and the evidence-base for their use is essentially unproven.

Perhaps the most high-profile use of management consultants in recent years came with their deployment into NHS organisations during the 2005/06 deficits crisis. Following an assessment by KPMG (ordered by the DH), private sector turnaround directors were appointed to each of the SHA regions in England, and dedicated 'turnaround teams' were sent by the DH into 18 NHS organisations (eight PCTs and ten NHS trusts) deemed to have the most severe financial problems.[a][8] Of this episode, which cost an estimated £22.1 million to the taxpayer,[9] the House of Commons Health Committee reported:

> We received mixed evidence regarding the effectiveness of turnaround teams. The teams themselves and the Department thought them value for money despite the high cost... [but] some witnesses were somewhat disparaging about their effectiveness.[10]

A proper assessment, however, was not carried out. The subsequent turnaround in NHS finances is presented as evidence of a positive effect, but the causal link is uncertain. It is almost impossible to assess effectiveness in the eight PCTs in receipt of turnaround teams, because all bar two have subsequently been involved in mergers. However, of the nine NHS trusts (excluding Hammersmith Hospital NHS Trusts, which has become part of Imperial Healthcare NHS Trust) three—Mid Yorkshire NHS Trust, Surrey and Sussex Healthcare NHS Trust and the Royal West Sussex NHS Trust—remained blacklisted as 'financially challenged' in the financial year 2007/08;[11] and none were rated better than 'fair' for use of resources by the Audit Commission.[12] One, Surrey and Sussex Healthcare NHS Trust—that has invested particularly heavily in management consultants—failed to meet seven out of 12 core standards relating to governance.[13]

The latest large-scale initiative is to bring management consultants into the commissioning process through the use of FESC. PCTs now have a list of 14 approved private sector organisations that they can use either to learn from or outsource elements of commissioning, such as assessment

---

(a) Subsequent reports, however, asserted that as many as a quarter, or 143, trusts actually received help from private sector turnaround teams before deficits were turned around. Triggle, N., 'Debt squads hit 25 per cent of trusts', *BBC News*, 13 November 2006.

and planning, contracting and procurement, settlement and review, performance management and patient/public engagement.[14] Yet there is little evidence that these outside organisations have a significantly better understanding of commissioning. In a *Health Service Journal* survey of 93 chief executives, commissioning directors, finance directors and others from a total of 74 PCTs, four in five thought there were ways other than FESC to help the commissioning process at PCT level, and nearly half thought that the framework would prove to be only 'a little' successful within their organisation.[15] Many, in particular, consider it to be overly bureaucratic and prescriptive. The first PCT to adopt FESC, Hillingdon, recently reported 'early indications are that it will not deliver projected savings', with the chair of its Audit Committee, Nigel Foxwell, saying: '... at this time [I cannot] see how these projects [will] result in value for money on performance to date'.[16] Despite this, the FESC programme was rolled out by the DH without the expected value for money analysis which, in the words of one FESC provider, was supposed to 'make sure it wasn't just a bonanza for the private sector'.[17] To be cynical, one can imagine difficulties in PCTs commissioning the private sector to commission for them if they aren't very good at commissioning themselves. Will programmes such as FESC succeed in building commissioning capacity and capability within PCTs; or will expenditure on FESC itself be seen as just another annual outlay?

The point is not that management consultants offer no value but that the circumstances around, and reasons for, their use should be carefully evaluated. In times of difficulty, if management consultants are hired it should be to complement, rather than substitute for, the more difficult but ultimately rewarding option of taking a long, hard look at one's organisation. The type of consultancy being used also matters. Those that talk the talk but ultimately only draw up endless master plans are much less likely to be effective than those that 'walk the territory', hear of important problems first hand and engage staff *à la* Gerry Robinson. It is only in such ways that learning will be retained and (hopefully) promulgated as part of healthcare delivery. As Jenny Simpson, chief executive of the British Association of Medical Managers (BAMM), has said: 'you can only change people's behaviour by making people want to do something. You have to be able to articulate a vision that presses an emotional button inside a person.'[18] For the management consultant, how to change culture permanently and ensure colleagues do not regress into the 'old comfort zone' remains the unanswerable question.[19]

Commandment Eight:
Love Your Bureaucracy

Bureaucracy is the art of making the possible impossible.

Javier Pascual Salcedo

Almost since the NHS's inception, cutting bureaucracy has been a theme of central government—and, of course, the opposition parties—yet no government has been particularly successful. New Labour's first significant act in power, the creation of Primary Care Groups to purchase health care, was justified at least partly on the basis of saving £1 billion in bureaucracy over five years.[1] Yet, wind on to 2004 and the Gershon Review found the DH could still oversee as much as £6.5 billion in 'efficiency savings' (more than any other government department);[2] John Reid, the then Secretary of State for Health, was announcing a bonfire of arms-length bodies to save some £500 million in bureaucracy;[3] and the internal market was back with a vengeance following the perceived failure of the initial reform programme.[4] Moving forward to 2008, the same theme emerged in Lord Darzi's report, which stated clearly: 'for those working in the NHS there is a need to reduce unnecessary bureaucracy, freeing up their time to care for patients'.[5] All the evidence suggests the bureaucracy that businesses in the NHS must deal with is as high, if not higher, than it has ever been.

The reasons for this are complex. Effective regulation, systemic processes and data collection are essential in any healthcare system. However, to be effective, it must be locally-owned and aligned to a purpose. Instead, much of the bureaucracy in the NHS can be seen as the result of the aforementioned trend towards the 'audit society' (see commandment two) and—to put it bluntly—the desire of the centre to maintain control. Here, the government has put

56

itself in a quandary. With NHS organisations increasingly shaped as businesses, but still operating in a single-payer system, there is neither direct control (as in line management to the DH) nor genuine consumer sovereignty. Organisations are neither accountable through traditional means to the state, nor directly to their customers (patients). In place of this catch-22, then, has come the rise of 'independent' regulators, either to 'guarantee' standards or as a new way to 'get things done' and force change.

However, while the responsibility for problems is shifted, the reality is that the reach and scope of government control is often either retained or increased. It is the state (via the NHS Appointments Commission) that typically appoints the boards of regulators and sets the focus of regulation as a whole. Most regulators are accountable to the government and/or DH.[6] What's more, with every re-organisation and policy review there tends to be a strengthening and/or extension of the regulatory framework, in order to implement, police and collect information on the recommendations, targets and initiatives deriving from them.[a]

(a) Roughly two thirds of the Healthcare Commission's Annual Health Check consists of looking at whether organisations have met government targets. For an example of the bureaucracy and regulation generated by policy reviews, we can take that carried out by Lord Darzi in 2008. At least eight new bodies are either created or confirmed as being created — the National Quality Board, SHA Quality Observatories, Health Innovation and Education Clusters, the NHS Leadership Council, the NHS Innovation Council (interim report), Medical Education England, Centre of Excellence and the Coalition for Better Health — alongside a whole host of initiatives including expanding the remit of NICE; a requirement on NHS (foundation) trusts to publish Quality Accounts and use Clinical Dashboards; the development of Commissioning for Quality and Innovation (CQUIN) and best

With such complex arrangements, flexibility is curbed (see commandment two) and, too often, the vital ingredient of trust goes out the window.

The bureaucratic burden—defined as the recurring costs of administrative activities that businesses are required to conduct in order to comply with the information obligations that are imposed through government or third-party regulation[7]—that NHS organisations now face is significant and onerous. The NHS Confederation[b] estimates that at least 69 bodies, from the new Care Quality Commission (CQC) to the Environment Agency, currently regulate, inspect, audit or demand information from NHS organisations—and this does not include core strategic NHS bodies such as SHAs and the DH.[8] To give an indication of the volume of work this generates, in 2004/05 the DH alone was responsible for around 600 data collections in the calendar year (some via SHAs), with the demands of others taking the total close to 1,000.[9]

This would be enough on its own, but the time taken complying with such requirements is multiplied by the

---

practice tariffs; enhancing NHS Choices to include more information on general practice; a commitment to personal care plans; the piloting of personal budgets and Integrated Care Organisations (ICOs); encouraging social enterprise; the introduction of a Leadership for Quality Certificate, Clinical Leadership Fellowships and a Clinical Management for Quality Programme; a tariff-based system for the training and education of clinicians; a re-invigoration of practice-based commissioning; and a reaffirmation of the extension of national regulation to cover general practice and to relate registration to healthcare acquired infections.

(b) The NHS Confederation is an independent membership body for the full range of organisations that make up the NHS.

uncoordinated nature of them. Regulators vary significantly in their statutory authority, powers, scope of action and approach. Some have general powers of enforcement (such as the Health and Safety Executive); some have specific powers relating to the NHS (such as the foundation trust regulator, Monitor). Some are public bodies (such as the National Audit Office, CQC and the Health Protection Agency); some are special health authorities (such as the National Patient Safety Agency and NICE); some are DH creations (such as the Cancer Peer Review) and some are generated by the NHS (such as the new National Quality Board). Most deal with a single facet of organisations, such as health and safety, medical education, professional standards *et cetera*, but some, such as the CQC and NICE, have more overarching roles.[10] There is now even a body, the CHRE, that is charged with 'ensuring consistency and good practice in healthcare regulation'—a regulator regulating the regulators, if you like.[11]

The mosaic such arrangements create for frontline organisations is, perhaps unsurprisingly, highly fragmented. Despite the efforts of initiatives such as the Concordat,[(c)] a large proportion of data requests received by NHS organisations are, in fact, for very similar information, just in different and incompatible formats. Little account is taken of the way in which data is collected, processed and recorded within them, with the net result that significant amounts of NHS resources are diverted to chasing information, re-

---

(c) The Concordat is a voluntary agreement between organisations that regulate, audit, inspect or review elements of health and health care in England. It was launched in June 2004 by ten organisations, led by the Healthcare Commission, with the aim of encouraging regulators to work together to co-ordinate their activities.

formatting data and preparing for an inspection. Looking at 35 of the bodies that can inspect or ask questions of healthcare providers, the NHS Confederation found that just four of the 77 standards laid out in the core operating document for NHS organisations *Standards for Better Health* are not duplicated. For five of the standards, ten or more bodies asked between 19 and 47 questions.[12] Such duplication is, again, only multiplied when requests from other NHS bodies, such as SHAs and PCTs in the case of NHS trusts, are factored in.

Individual clinicians find themselves in no less onerous a position. In 2004 a consultant surgeon, who is also an academic, listed the bodies to which he had to report. They included: eight national bodies, starting with the GMC; eight hospital bodies, ranging from the Clinical Governance Committee to the Pre-Registration House Officer and Senior House Officer Reviews for the Post-Graduate Team; and six university bodies, including the Annual University Appraisal and the Research Governance Committee.[13] In primary care, every GP must now complete the 135 or so boxes required by the QOF, proving they have—or justifying why they have not—followed the recommended course of treatment for each patient with a chronic disease.

A further trick is for government to change the regulatory climate just as regulators are getting used to working with each other, and NHS organisations are getting used to, and have calibrated their systems, to work with them. For example the QOF, despite having been relatively effective in its aim of raising biomedical quality, is now being brought under the remit of NICE.[14(d)] Since being founded in

---

(d) We have chosen not to mention the QOF's unintended consequences here, which have been significant (see commandment five).

November 1999, the Commission for Health Improvement (CHI) became the Healthcare Commission in 2004, and is now—along with the Commission for Social Care Inspection (CSCI) and the Mental Health Act Commission—being subsumed into a 'super-regulator', the Care Quality Commission (CQC). The transition has already been uncomfortable, with the handover rated as 'red risk' by the Healthcare Commission in February 2009,[15] but further problems are likely. With extended powers of enforcement (including issuing financial penalty notices and suspending the registration of an organisation), the CQC has defined its mission as not just to set, monitor and enforce minimum standards, but also to drive improvements in the quality of care. It is, therefore, difficult to see how it will not clash with other regulators, such as NICE, the National Quality Board and Monitor, that also have a stake in this field. The conclusions of the NHS Confederation in 2007 that 'the present regulatory processes are piecemeal, complex [and] confused, being made up of many different bodies who [sic] hold different statuses... and have different powers to control behaviour' are just as true today.[16]

No-one quite knows how much all this costs businesses in the NHS in terms of time, resources and attention pulled from patient care, but it is significant. To take a particular example, it is estimated that the administration associated with the QOF can alone take up to 20-30 hours per week for the average practice, including 2-3 hours of clinical time. While some of this is beneficial to patients—it tends to encourage a more accurate and active monitoring of long-term conditions—much data collection is not. In one survey conducted in 2003, managers of secondary care organisations considered that 58 per cent of information collected could not be used for any internal purpose.[17]

There is little doubt that this has contributed to a significant rise in non-clinical costs. Over the past ten years, the number of managers and senior managers in NHS organisations has increased by 64.6 per cent, compared with 42.4 per cent for doctors and 25.3 per cent for nurses, until the total number of managers, administrators and clerks (207,778) now exceeds the number of beds (167,019).[18] Management costs—though falling as an overall proportion of the NHS budget—rose from £1,728 million in 1997/8 to £2,287 million in 2003/4.[19] And, in early 2009, the Conservative Party estimated that funding for the DH, its quangos and regional authorities—none of whom deliver frontline care—had reached more than £12 billion, a 103 per cent increase since 2003.[20]

Meetings and committees that draw up plans unlikely to go anywhere, or severely over-complicate those that should, are commonplace. Clinicians, if they are not careful, can end up spending more time sitting on these than treating patients. The development of the National Service Framework (NSF) for Older People is one such example. Focused on stroke, it effectively mirrored guidance already detailed in a comprehensive document by the Royal College of Physicians. Despite this, the NSF took two years to produce, predominantly due to the number of recommendations the minister would allow the working party to make; which aspects should be thrown out (none); how the document should be structured; and the continual change of administrative personnel that held veto power, but were ignorant of clinical matters.[21] Rules and routines too easily become more important than the ends they were designed to serve.

The NHS would do well to look at things the other way around. Bureaucracy should never act as a barrier to businesses and people serving patients better. While regulation is necessary, the focus should be on what makes effective regulation, rather than simply upping the volume and scope in the hope of 'enforcing' standards. Regulators may well have good intentions, but how they go about their business may actually have a negative impact on those delivering care. For every expense incurred, every department created, every project taken on, a basic question should be asked: will this help patients? If the answer is not a ringing and positive 'yes', we would do well to ask why it is there at all.[22]

Commandment Nine:
Send Mixed Messages

The single biggest problem in communication is the illusion that it has taken place.

George Bernard Shaw

World-class organisations, both within and outside the health sector, base their strategy on a clear vision that unites and guides employees towards providing the best service possible. Employees know what the priorities are, know where they stand, and are able to use this to work out what to do in the situations they encounter.

In industry, Disney is the archetypal example of such an approach. As of 2008 it maintained its position as number one in *Fortune Magazine's* 'most admired entertainment industry' category, was ranked number three across all US companies for people management, and remains one of the top companies in the world in terms of customer satisfaction.[1] Key to Disney's success is the clarity of its vision: 'safety, courtesy, the show and efficiency'. All members of Disney's 'cast' from street sweepers to managers attend the Disney University to grow into the organisation's culture, thereby creating a sense of value, pride and purpose (around five per cent of the organisation's revenue is spent on training).[2] The words 'it's not my job' are forbidden. Instead, all staff are encouraged to 'dream, believe, dare and do'. Disney's philosophy is based on a belief that the best ideas are generated by those closest to the frontline, that each time a frontline employee's idea is used, a culture of creativity and innovation is reinforced.[3]

The same clarity of vision and sense of worth is vital in health care, particularly in facilitating effective leadership and teamwork.[4] One theme running throughout this book has been the importance of change and quality improvement being 'owned' by those on the frontline. Equally important, however, is that the same motives are held and expressed by senior managers, clinicians and chief executives. Quality (except in a very haphazard form) will seldom improve in a business when the actions or words or those at the top do not support it.[5] As Paul Bate and colleagues concluded from their pioneering work tracking the improvement journeys of nine leading hospitals in Europe and the USA:

> Quality is often presented in the literature as a scientific method or discipline, but it is as much a question of value orientation and outlook.
>
> We should perhaps be spending more time developing professional and corporate commitment than directly trying to improve quality: programmes or projects quickly run out of energy; being professional is a lifelong vocation and the very fuel of giving service.[6]

A particularly interesting example of this in action is the Griffin Hospital in Connecticut, USA, which, under the management of its chief executive Patrick Charmel, achieved notable results through actively applying 'Disney-like' principles. In 1980, 30 per cent of the local community said they would avoid the hospital at all costs; it was struggling financially; and on every measure was the worst in the area. Charmel then invoked a strategy based on employee pride as a roadmap to patient satisfaction. Most important in this was mandatory training to orientate staff to the hospital's vision—Quality and Service, Respect and Dignity, Collaboration, Entrepreneurship and Innovation and Stewardship[7]—and using simulations to place them in the experience of being a patient. With a resolute focus on patient care from the patient's perspective, Griffin Hospital started the walk along the 'punishing terrain' of improvement. There were no mixed messages. In 2008, the hospital's patient satisfaction rates were over 95 per cent and, remarkably for a hospital, it is now ranked in the top 100 companies in the USA to work for.[8]

The Luther Midelfort Compact

What can you expect from our group?

1. A physician-led organisation that manages with integrity, honesty and open communication

2. A commitment to recruit and retain superior physicians and staff

3. Provide support to physicians and departments as they strive to accomplish organisational goals

4. A commitment to make the changes needed to ensure future success.

What can our group expect from you?

1. A focus on decision-making that serves the needs of our patients and their families

2. A commitment to treat all members of Luther Midelfort with respect and embrace a team approach to achieving optimal patient care

3. A commitment to professional development including:

   a) Current knowledge within an individual's area of expertise

   b) Use of objective measures of clinical outcome to improve care given to our patients

4. A recognition that personal change will be needed to accomplish organisational goals.

Source: Bate, P., Mendel, P. and Robert, G., (2008)

Other healthcare organisations have gone one step further and sought to embed the organisation's vision in staff contracts. The Luther-Midelfort Mayo Clinic, which won the Acclaim Award in 2005 (the American Medical Group Association's most prestigious award conferred to only one recipient per year), has a physician compact that is used to develop a high degree of organisational identity and commitment among physicians to its goals, mission and vision.

Among NHS organisations, there are similar examples of such commitment. At Royal Devon and Exeter NHS Foundation Trust, Bate and colleagues trace the story of high quality care, highlighting: 'the distinct importance of organisational identity... the collective self-definitions of an organisation and the groups within it of "who we are", the collective role "we" play, the distinctive characteristics "we" possess, and the image "we" wish to project'.[9] Feelings of solidarity have acted as a powerful catalyst for collective action and enabled the trust to embrace a more organic—as opposed to a strict command-and-control—approach to quality improvement. Organisational structure is flat and the senior management team are accessible, open and willing to 'walk the talk'. Quality is framed specifically in terms of patient care: 'My philosophy is let's be clear about why patients come to this organisation', said its chief executive. 'It's because GPs believe we have clinicians who are good: they don't come because I, or the trust board, are here.'[10]

However, the same clarity of vision is not in evidence across the NHS. Too often mixed messages prevail. While 79 per cent of the 290,000 NHS staff surveyed by the Healthcare Commission in 2008 said they knew their responsibilities, only 65 per cent said they had clear objectives. Only 55 per cent said they knew how their role contributed to what their trust was trying to achieve; just 47 per cent believed their trust communicates clearly on these aims (21 per cent said they did not); and just 39 per cent felt that they worked in well-structured teams in which staff had clear objectives, worked closely together to meet these objectives, and regularly reviewed and reflected on performance.[11] Some of this reflects internal problems, but the impact of the external environment should not be underestimated. As the NHS Operating Framework for 2009/10 acknowledges: 'local initiative has all too often been stifled in the past by heavy-handed bureaucracy or mixed and contradictory messages'.[12]

The irony, however, is that one need look no further than the same document for a microcosm of this. In its attempt to draw together existing national priorities, the recommendations of Lord Darzi's *Next Stage Review,* the world class commissioning assurance regime and many other disparate initiatives into a coherent framework, the Operating Framework is full of double-binds. The Framework insists that 'improvements in quality cannot be driven from Whitehall',[13] yet in practice reads as a shopping list of demands on SHAs, PCTs and provider organisations—from the 21 existing targets (now labelled 'commitments') and five national priorities (with their 64 associated 'vital signs') to the development of Quality Accounts. Phrases such as '[PCTs] will want to', 'need to' or 'should seek to' are the words of choice. More specifically, the existing national priorities and Lord Darzi's reforms sit side by side, but are not integrated in any real sense. The idea, for example, that money spent on developing Quality Accounts, new data systems and paying for for better outcomes through the Commissioning for Quality and Innovation (CQUIN) scheme—all reforms proposed by Lord Darzi—will mean less money to spend on meeting national priorities or service development is not tackled.[14]

The danger of such incoherence, if not already evident, is made abundantly clear by the Windmill simulations carried out by the King's Fund in 2007. 'There is no way of working out where all the changes will lead', complained PCTs, hospital trusts, the independent sector and regulators, 'there is no "big picture".'[15] On the one hand, organisations are supposed to be businesses operating in a competitive market and focused on customers; on the other central targets are set and ministerial rhetoric still holds organisations responsible for stability in the local health economy. What, for example, are PCTs, that have the goals of world class commissioning as their core business plan, to make of all the initiatives listed above?[16] This, the King's Fund concluded, 'is making managers and decision-makers less certain about where to make their long-term investments and disinvestments'.[17]

More importantly, such mixed messages also make it remarkably difficult for those in charge of businesses in the NHS to define and embed a core vision around patient care. Some do, but too many don't. In all the trusts investigated by the Healthcare Commission for poor standards of care there is a common theme: a poor track record of dealing with conflicting priorities manifesting itself in a 'vulnerability to being consumed by the business of healthcare, in the form of mergers, reconfiguration of services, financial deficits and targets'.[18] Successful businesses focus on the end goal: providing high quality services for patients.

Commandment Ten:
Be Afraid of the Future

We are all in the gutter, but some of us are looking at stars.

Oscar Wilde

The NHS's history has coincided with the triumph of modern medicine. Joint replacements; coronary artery by-pass grafts; minimally invasive surgery; day surgery; home-based hospital care; CT and MRI scanning; catheterisation; drugs for infections, high blood pressure, hypertension and raised cholesterol were nowhere to be seen in 1948, but are now standard practice.

There is nothing to suggest the next 60 years will be different; medicine has not, as the social historian Roy Porter put it, 'accomplished its mission'. At the most basic level, there are many unrealised opportunities to apply scientific understanding to new ways of preventing, postponing and treating disease, and to make sure new technologies are universally available to people who need them. Again and again researchers find that the 'rule of halves' still very much applies: half of those who have the risk factor (such as high blood pressure) are not aware of it; half of those in whom it is detected are not treated; and half of those who are treated are not treated adequately.[1] To add to the continuum, disruptive innovations will enable things that could be done by only highly-qualified specialists a few years ago to be done by newly-qualified nurses, or even patients.[2] And health services research, particularly when purposely linked to clinical care in as close to real time as possible, has much to offer in providing the quality improvement tools to deliver health care in the optimum way.[3]

70

It is also possible—and even likely—that medical science, having now taken off, is on something of an exponential learning curve. Cancer care, to take one example, is being revolutionised. The availability of real-time verification systems and image guided radiotherapy can now target tumours without laying waste to surrounding tissue; PET–CT and other imaging techniques are being used not just to plan radical treatment but also to monitor tumour destruction during therapy; and around 50 new drug applications will be made in the next few years for molecularly targeted anti-cancer (or 'smart') drugs [4] All are truly remarkable advances in medical science that draw on fundamental physics, physical chemistry, biochemistry, physiology, pharmacology, and a whole series of modern industrial techniques, clinical trials and service-line innovations.[5]

Yet, in the NHS and the field of health care generally, pessimism tends to reign: we are as much the victims of 'the failures of the successes' of medicine as the beneficiaries of its wonders. How are we to afford all these expensive drugs and technologies that are keeping old people older for longer? Three points should be made here. First, the problem may not be as acute as we think. The ability of medicine to keep people alive for longer does not necessarily mean they will be ill for longer and cost the health system more. The vast majority of people in fact enjoy resonably good health in later life, and there is little evidence that medical care in the last year of life is becoming more aggressive or technological.[6] Second, while new technology unquestionably drives up costs in the short-term, there is equally huge potential for disruptive innovation to enable health systems to deliver existing medical care at much lower cost (think how much cheaper DVD players are now than when they first came out).[7] Third, certain new technologies and drugs

71

do, in fact, have only marginal effects on health and well-being *vis-à-vis* less 'scientific' interventions, such as improving the humanity and appropriateness of care. Would it, in the case of these technologies, be unreasonable for a public health system to accept the realities of a finite budget and support supplementary forms of payment for these treatments, such as insurance packages and voluntarism?[8]

Instead of a more rational and optimistic response, however, fear of 'the future', namely, how the NHS budget will cover the health care people demand, tends to set government in a frenzy. Initiative after initiative is tried in the hope that one of the potpourri will, to pilfer the words of Sheila Leatherman and Kim Sutherland, 'be infused with magical powers... and slay the bad performance monster'.[9] These may be grouped under three broad themes: to control costs so that people consume less health care; to control reimbursement and uphold 'national standards' in order to 'force' providers to become more 'efficient'; and to divert resources to areas deemed to be priority cases (more often than not those where patient advocacy groups are most effective at focusing media attention).[a] As we have seen throughout the commandments, the result of such strategy tends to be paradoxical. Though it is not a zero-sum game, as the state has intervened in more and more branches of health care, the ability and inclination of businesses (and individuals) at the coal face to drive improvement has been curbed; and, perversely, inefficiency is actually locked in rather than driven out. Cultures of fear and blame too easily

---

(a) Much less is said of the so-called 'Cinderella' services that provide for the elderly, chronically ill and psychiatric patients, where so many already turn to the private sector to provide care.

replace those of ingenuity and success. Far from sending out messages of trust and support, the government actually encourages patients to be suspicious of clinicians' motives.[b]

This atmosphere inevitably permeates patient care. Chief executives and managers who are reluctant to do anything too radical for fear of being accused of 'rocking the boat',[10] and clinicians who fear they are neglecting patient care by inadvertently focusing on targets and initiatives,[11] do not make for happy patients. The pressures of day-to-day practice and the inherent uncertainties in medicine mean Hippocrates's great injunction 'first, do no harm' is surprisingly difficult to follow even in a positive environment conducive to high quality care—let alone one that is not. As is being increasingly recognised in health services research, safety and quality (as in other industries) is not just a function of the skills of individual clinicians and mangers, but also of the organisational, systemic and cultural environment in which they are working.[12] The doctor/patient relationship, for example, is influenced by all manner of things, from the content of the consultation and a positive interaction between values and beliefs held by the doctor and patient to anything influencing the *context* of that consultation, such as incentive structures, policy, regulation, finance and HR.[13] When this context is permeated by a fear of the future, negative energy and incoherent strategy, patient care—particularly the human side of it—will suffer, even if clinicians are loath to admit it. The reality is that doctors and nurses, who may well have between a quarter

---

(b) The NHS Constitution, billed as enshrining the principles and values of the NHS, was recently sold as ending the era of 'the doctor knows best'.

and half a million appointments in the course of a 40-year career, have to exhibit almost superhuman empathy and attentiveness if they are not going to appear apathetic or even inhumane.

There is however a deeper risk in all this: that clinicians in particular start to believe the myth that they are 'forever' condemned to mistrust and powerlessness. As Dr Mike Dixon, chair of the NHS Alliance, has said: the disease in NHS organisations is that we have very motivated doctors saying they think this or that is the right thing to do, but ultimately concluding the system is such they couldn't possibly risk doing it.[14] Clinician-led advances, particularly those that 'sneak in from below' and overtake existing ways of doing things, have become increasingly difficult to implement.[15] The care of disorders which primarily involve one system in the body—from ear-ache to cardiac and renal illnesses—will, for example, probably migrate to focused institutions whose scope enables them to provide better care with less complexity-driven overheads. Many clinicians see huge potential in building integrated networks across primary and secondary care to support this. The field of patient safety is also awash with pioneering ideas. The use of After Action Review and variable hierarchies to learn from mistakes and 'near misses';[16] innovative anti-bullying schemes; and learning from techniques like standard operating procedures used in 'high reliability' fields (such as Formula 1 and aviation) are just a few coming on-stream.[17] But too many ideas, as we saw in commandment one, remain bubbling beneath the surface.[18] In 2008, only 66 per cent of NHS staff felt they were able to contribute towards improvements at work.[19]

This need not be so. Clinicians and patients alike must be able to see opportunity, not paralysis; solutions, not just problems; vision, not confusion. The future should be looked at with optimism, not fear. Real progress should be about creating cultures that enable new ideas to burst through the surface; where the search is for ways of eliminating risks associated with new technologies and ways of working, rather than seeing the obstacles as insurmountable. Real progress should be about trusting frontline staff to bring a smile to patients' faces, to value the power of anxiety lessened, and to value the power of questions answered and expectations met. 'How wonderful' as the diarist Anne Frank wrote, 'is [it] that nobody need wait a single moment before starting to improve the world.'

Commandment Eleven:
Lose Passion for Work and Life

If you want people to do a good job, give them a good job to do

Frederick Herzberg

It is a peculiar feature of the NHS that few who work in it, or with it, describe themselves as happy. Pharmaceutical companies, manufacturers of medical devices and innovators of technology are frustrated, for, despite introducing life-saving drugs, treatments, therapies and devices, they get blamed for driving up costs and are vilified for their profit motives. Managers are stressed about bureaucratic burdens, about the ironically termed 'redisorganisation' of NHS structures,[1] and fear being blamed for things that are their responsibility, but which they struggle to do anything about.[2] The government, for its part, finds itself in the impossible position of running one of the largest organisations (or collection of organisations) on the planet and being criticised whenever anything goes wrong.

The greatest dissatisfaction, however, is found in the medical and nursing professions. To be sure, they can be a troublesome bunch, sometimes guilty of directing the media searchlight to advertise their own grievances.[3] As a rule, they are also quite conservative; nailed to what philosophers have called the 'natural standpoint'. However, in a labour-intensive industry like health care, doctors, nurses and health professionals are the key resource—managerially as well as clinically. The best of the work businesses in the NHS do is achieved by the professionalism of the clinical staff working in them. Medicine is a complex job in terms of the amount of information that must be grasped to practice effectively; in terms of the amount of emotional load doctors and nurses are asked to carry—their own and their

76

patients'—and in terms of workload and time pressures. It should always be remembered that physicians, in particular, often work on the margins of knowledge and bear a heavy burden of responsibility in difficult circumstances. Uncertainty becomes an agony of decision, and errors of omission and commission may haunt one for years— notwithstanding the risk of clinical negligence cases, GMC hearings and being pilloried in the press.[4] In 2008, 66 per cent of staff in acute trusts reported regularly doing unpaid overtime, and countless reports point to abnormally high levels of stress and sickness absence.[5] *Per se*, medicine and nursing needs resillent people to survive in it.

This, however, tends to be accepted by those entering the profession. The root cause of dissatisfaction is not so much the stresses of the job, but that structural change in the NHS over the past 30 years—despite introducing business-like principles—has typically served to increase this burden by wresting control of the service from those who are delivering it. Any job, as Adrian Kenny put it, is a balance of satisfaction, salary and support.[6] Doctors can no longer complain about their salaries (though many nurses may be entitled to) and the practice of medicine is intrinsically satisfying, both in terms of the interest in medicine itself, and in terms of the range of people it allows you to meet. It is support that tends to be lacking: a culture, if you like, of warm applause, of encouraging quality improvement. The former editor of the *British Medical Journal*, Richard Smith, summarises this well:

> The most obvious cause of doctors' unhappiness is that they feel overworked and under-supported. They hear politicians make extravagant promises but then must explain to patients why the health service cannot deliver what is promised. Endless initiatives are announced, but on the ground doctors find that operating lists are cancelled, they cannot admit or discharge patients, and community services are disappearing. They struggle to respond,

but they feel as though they are battling the system rather than being supported by it.[7]

The current editor, Fiona Godlee, has gone a step further, saying that 'the spirit of medical professionalism is quietly dying'.[8] In conversation and in print, clinicians in every business and at every level of the service complain of a lack of respect, understanding and trust.[9] In a survey by *Hospital Doctor* magazine in 2007 of over 1,400 GPs and hospital doctors, 69 per cent said they would not recommend a career in medicine, with 54 per cent rating their morale as 'poor' or 'terrible'.[10] The root of the problem is not a declining attraction to medicine, or a decline in the desire to 'make a difference', it is the grip of central control that—while recognising that there is unacceptable and arrogant practice out there—too often prevents doctors providing the best care they know.[a] A survey of staff working in NHS organisations by the Healthcare Commission in 2006 found that only two-fifths were able to answer positively to the question: 'As a patient of this trust, I would be happy with the standard of care provided'.[11] Later, in 2007, staff in acute trusts were asked whether 'care of patients/service users is my trust's top priority'. Only 48 per cent agreed, 23 per cent disagreed and 28 per cent sat on the fence, neither agreeing nor disagreeing.[12] In 2008, job satisfaction had improved slightly, but still only 60 per cent said they were 'satisfied

---

(a) In 2007, a poll carried out by doctors.net, Britain's busiest medical website, revealed a profession disillusioned with central diktat and angered by the growth of bureaucracy. Of the respondents, more than two fifths were young and had graduated since 2000. Fifty-six per cent said there'd been no improvement in the NHS since 2002; 72 per cent said they didn't think the extra money had been well spent; 72 per cent said there'd been no improvement in quality of care.

with the quality of work and patient care they were able to deliver', and just 52 per cent said they would recommend their trust as a place to work.[13]

This matters, both for the health of staff, and for their patients.[14] Clinicians and managers are human beings; a cheerful and well motivated staff will inevitably deliver a better quality of service to patients. Without this, enthusiasm for really engaging with patients tends to go. Demoralised doctors tend to quietly acquiesce and stop thinking it worthwhile to argue their corner, or will only do it to score off someone, rather than with a proper focus on improving patient care. 'Nothing great in the world', as the philosopher Georg Friedrich Hegel once said, 'has been accomplished without passion.' The patient is seen and treated but will feel like a number, rather than a person. Worse, irritability tends to breed mistakes; relevant information is not gathered or, if gathered, its significance is not realised.[15] While doctors need routines and automatic pilot to get safely through the complexities of medicine, anyone who allows this to dull their vigilance will soon be punished as the unusual presentation is missed or the signal is lost in the noise.[16]

Medicine, the profession of making sick people better, should kindle the ultimate fire of enthusiasm. Yet the basic feeling of too many doctors and nurses is that they are good at their jobs despite the NHS and the businesses they are working for, not because of them. How many clinicians have found themselves uttering the words: 'that's good enough', that's not my job', 'I don't care' or 'I'm retiring anyway'. If they are, businesses will more than likely be failing, and will probably be failing patients too. But give the same clinicians (and, for that matter, managers) ownership; something to be passionate about; an emotional connection once more with people, organisations and dreams, not statistics, bureaucracy and targets—and see what might happen.

Conclusion

In her Reith Lectures in 2002, the philosopher Onora O'Neill argued: 'if we want a culture of public service, professional and public servants must, in the end, be free to serve the public rather than their paymasters'.[1] It is, in a sense, a no-brainer; as a public service, the NHS is there to provide the best possible care to the public and to its patients—not the government, the Department of Health or the NHS Executive. Yet, presiding over a monopoly of funding, resource allocation and provision, the latter have historically found it impossible not to meddle; and frontline organisations have consequently found it impossible not to first look up for direction rather than focus their energies squarely the needs of patients. The historic error has been to conflate the need for collective choices and collective action with central direction and political control.

The idea behind introducing market incentives and setting NHS organisations up as businesses was, then, to try to engineer a sea-change in this standpoint; to re-focus attention on meeting the needs of the public and patients; and to create a marketplace for entrepreneurs. Increased autonomy would result in an end to direct line management by the DH. If organisations then failed to serve the public (or at least their patients) well, they would not just have unhappy patients, but would more than likely start to lose custom too. The reality, however, has been very different.

Being rigidly 'designed', directed and regulated, many features of the market that has emerged have made important aspects of patient care, such as collaborative working and the delivery of genuinely integrated care, more rather than less difficult. Increasingly devolved and autonomous structures may be in place, and government may have stepped back from the *day-to-day* running of the service, but initiatives, targets and policy reviews ensure

80

that the centre still calls the shots. Where power of government has genuinely been rescinded, a new breed of 'independent' regulators has proved more than happy to take up the mantle. In essence, there is a profound contradiction at the heart of the NHS: organisations are now supposed to be acting like businesses in the sense of streamlining and tailoring services to 'win' customers (patients), yet they are still forced to face towards the state — they have to, because this is where the funding and ultimate power lies.

The toxicity of this mix is there for all to see: managers, clinicians, health professionals and, increasingly, patients do not know where to turn. Fledgling businesses in the NHS have tried to put patients first, and some have shown signs of success — the Central Middlesex Hospital, recently showcased by the NHS Confederation;[2] UCLH NHS Foundation Trust's planned Cancer Centre, where each floor is to be designed around the needs of patients with different cancers;[3] and Ealing PCT's 'Patient Experience Tracker'[4] are a few examples. Yet all they know for certain is that if the Secretary of State for Health issues edicts such as a deep-clean of hospitals, an 18-week waiting time target or no more mixed wards, they must follow or face the consequences. The aforementioned historic error is being repeated, just in a different form. The priorities of businesses are forced into being profoundly different from those of their patients: concerned with conforming to processes and meeting central targets, than with people and the illnesses they have.

In this unfortunate situation, it is the very building block of medicine, the interaction between clinician and patient, that — somewhat ironically — has been most neglected. The consultation has been described in many ways, but the most recent epithet is 'beleaguered'.[5] Time and resource constraints; indecisive management; additional bureaucratic tasks; a lack of continuity; and above all a lack of tolerance and trust, are hindering the ability of clinicians to perform their most basic tasks: to listen, analyse symptoms and to care.[6] The careful observation, stabilisation and treatment of the patient presenting in A&E with severe asthma, or optimum treatment for the patient presenting in general practice with complex co-morbidities, comes at the risk of irritating government through missing targets. Quality improvement and the development of new ideas are simult-aneously encouraged and suppressed, and proper eval-uation of the results becomes difficult if not irrelevant.

The critical point is this: 'autonomy' means nothing if all it is used for is finding more innovative ways of meeting central requirements. In essence this is why, acknowledging there are nuances particular to each commandment and exceptions to every rule, we find businesses in the NHS are keeping Keough's 'ten commandments': they tend to be risk-averse; inflexible, bureaucratic and increasingly isolated from their patients; playing the game close to the foul line; and afraid of the future. They are inclined to dance to the tune of their shareholders and boards of directors (the government, Department of Health and NHS Executive), rather than focus on customers (patients) and what they need. Patients are too often put to the back, rather than the forefront, of thinking, the opposite of what a market-driven system should tend to inspire.

But, enough negativity. We have a diagnosis, what of the cure? For this, we would do well to start with the wisdom of the President of the Institute for Healthcare Improvement, Donald Berwick: 'Looking', he said, 'is not seeing. Listening is not hearing. It is possible to miss so much that is right in front of us if we lack the categories and skills to notice.'[7] To put it another way, you can, as the former government minister Lord Peyton once said, 'know the shape of the forest, but have no idea what is going on under the trees'.[8] We have unwittingly reached a point in the NHS where blind faith in structures and processes—important though they are—has made businesses (and the government) immune to what is actually happening on the ground, where the world of people, cultures and emotion make the real difference. Staff have become experts in running systems and massaging figures that provide chief executives, board directors, civil servants and politicians with exactly the data and information they need to satisfy themselves that all is well, but do they bear any relation to reality? If the cases of Mid Staffordshire NHS Foundation Trust and Birmingham Children's Hospital NHS Foundation Trust are anything to go by, we should be sceptical: you can tick all the boxes but still provide a woefully inadequate service.

Despite all the reforms and additional money poured into the organisation, the NHS and the businesses that now make it up are essentially unreformed in terms of hearts and minds and clinical structures. People—the ones who actually deliver the service—have been the neglected element. Caring, compassion, ingenuity and a desire to 'make a difference' are still out there, but have too easily been paralysed in a system that prefers to over-estimate the importance of legislation and regulation as markers of success and under-estimate local power to drive quality. It is like being caught in quicksand: the harder one struggles, the faster one disappears from view. Businesses—operating in a system dominated by such thinking—have typically either failed to grasp that command-and-control is not the answer or have failed to match rhetoric with reality. The prevailing culture is one of blame and fear, rather than openness and optimism.

The world's leading businesses such as Coca-Cola, Apple, Disney and Toyota, and the world's top hospitals such as the

Griffin Hospital, the Mayo Clinic and the Johns Hopkins Health System, do things very differently. They do not begin with a desire to meet diktats, targets and central initiatives. Instead, they begin with a clear understanding of what their customers and patients want and need, and develop services accordingly.[9] In doing so they pay huge attention to building emotional connections in staff; to conveying a clear vision; to building relationships; to giving staff scope for action; and, above all, to offering them the opportunity to be a part of something that inspires. It is not easy, and developing supportive cultures takes time. But top organisations recognise that when a business loses the energies of its staff and becomes distracted by internal issues, it will start to deliver a poor service to its customers (read patients).

What would this mean for the NHS? In essence that businesses shift their focus to answering two simple questions: 'what are patients' wants and needs?' and 'how do we get clinicians (and patients) to work more effectively together to meet them?'. For clinicians and clinical leaders, this means stepping up to the plate to drive quality improvement, and modernising working practices to deliver the right things to patients. For managers, this means encouraging pluralism, understanding the dynamics of the interaction between clinicians and patients and appreciating that the spreadsheet does not reveal all. For patients this means getting the help, advice and treatment they need accurately and accessibly.[a][10] And across the board it means developing cultures that back innovation and success.[b]

(a) Ultimately, we might expect patients to become what Julian Tudor-Hart has described as 'co-producers of their own health' or what J.A. Muir Gray has called 'resourceful'. Taking the tablets may be part of the treatment, but as medicine advances patients will need

The ability of people and frontline organisations to do this, however, depends on one crucial thing: that government and regulatory bodies grasp the implications of a more entrepreneurial, organic, way of working, and allow businesses and individuals to be change-makers and shakers. As a market, and a collection of businesses, the NHS should have real potential to deliver benefits to patients, but as yet we simply do not know if this is the case: it has not been allowed to work.[c] It is no good preaching one thing and practicing another. The government must make some serious choices. Does it want a market, or a centralised monopoly? Does it want businesses or 'arms-length' bodies of the state? Does it want a culture based on trust, or on

---

to engage with their doctors and negotiate solutions that work for them. Many patients want more responsibility, both in decision-making and the management of disease.

(b) This, too, is where the power of having a market in the NHS should kick in. The principle advantage of such a structure is often misunderstood. It is less that markets bring about a 'perfect' allocation of resources, more that they encourage a pluralistic environment that—in the context of health care—grants autonomy to professionals to try to serve patients better. Having a multiplicity of businesses permits numerous small-scale experiments in how to improve the service on offer, rather than a single, large-scale one in the case of monopoly. Through patients being able to choose between them, the successful experiment is quickly imitated, while the unsuccessful quickly folds. People and businesses are encouraged to innovate and adopt flexibility, rather than conservatism, as a natural standpoint.

(c) There is, of course, an ongoing debate, referred to in the introduction, as to whether markets can be truly effective in a single-payer (tax-funded) structure. For now, we say only this: the bureaucratic wish for standardisation and control is the antithesis of any market-like system.

hefty regulation? The current morass is suiting no-one, least of all patients. There is a wealth of new ideas and untapped energy for good amongst those who use and work for NHS organisations. They need a clear vision.

Notes

Preface

1   Keough, D., *The Ten Commandments for Business Failure*, London: Penguin Books, 2008, p. 178.

Introduction

1   Watkin, B., *The National Health Service: The First Phase 1948-1974 and After*, London: George Allen & Unwin, 1978, p. 40

2   Klein, R., *The New Politics of the NHS: from creation to reinvention* (5th edn), Oxford: Radcliffe Medical Publishing, 2006.

3   Quoted in Timmins, N., 'Challenges of private provision in the NHS', *BMJ*, 2005;331:1193-1195.

4   Hunter, D.J., *The Health Debate*, Bristol: Policy Press, 2008; Tudor-Hart, J., *The Political Economy of Health care: a clinical perspective*, Bristol: Policy Press, 2006; Leatherman, S. and Sutherland, K., *The Quest for Quality: Refining the NHS Reforms*, London: The Nuffield Trust, 2008.

5   Kay, J., *The Truth about Markets*, London: Penguin Books, 2003.

6   Keough, D., *The Ten Commandments for Business Failure*, New York: Penguin Books, 2008.

7   Patel, A. and Ingleton, R., 'Apple's way will bear most fruit', *HSJ*, 15 January 2009, p. 16.

8   Harvey, S., Liddell, A. and McMahon, L., *Windmill 2007: the future of healthcare reforms in England*, London: The King's Fund, 2007; Curry, N., Goodwin, N., Naylor, C. and Robertson, R., *Practice-based Commissioning. Reinvigorate, Replace or Abandon?* London: The King's Fund, 2008.

9   Institute for Fiscal Studies, 'Budget Analysis 2009'; http://www.ifs.org.uk/projects/304
NHS Confederation, 'Dealing with the downturn: the greatest ever leadership challenge for the NHS', London: NHS Confederation, 2009.

NHS plc

1 Klein, R., *The New Politics of the NHS: from creation to reinvention* (5th edn), Oxford: Radcliffe Medical Publishing, 2006.

2 Pollock, A., *NHS Plc: the privatisation of our health care*, London: Verso Books, 2004.

3 See:
http://www.dh.gov.uk/en/FreedomOfInformation/Freedomofinfor
mationpublicationschemefeedback/FOIreleases/DH_4109504

4 Monitor, *About Monitor: effective regulation, better patient care*, London: Monitor, 2007.

5 Ham, C., 'World class commissioning: a health policy chimera?'. *J Health Serv Res Policy*, 2008;13;2.

6 See:
http://www.dh.gov.uk/en/managingyourorganisation/commissioni
ng/worldclasscommissioning/index.htm

7 Hawkes, N., 'Analysis: a classier NHS, but choice still an illusion', *The Times*, 1 July 2008.

8 Department of Health, *The NHS in England: the operating framework for 2008/09*, London: TSO, 2008.

9 Darzi, A., *High Quality Care for All: NHS next stage review final report*, London: TSO, 2008, p. 5.

10 Department of Health, *Consultation on a Regime for Unsustainable NHS Providers*, London: TSO, 2008.

11 Department of Health, *Delivering Investment in General Practice: implementing the new GMS contract*, London: TSO, 2003.

12 Ellins, J., Ham, C. and Parker, H., 'Opening up the primary care market', *BMJ* 2009;338:b1127.

13 Carvel, J., 'Patients to rate and review their GPs on NHS website', *Guardian*, 30 December 2008.

14 Pollock, *NHS Plc*; Tallis, R., *Hippocratic Oaths: medicine and its discontents*, London: Atlantic Books, 2004.

15 Kay, J., *The Truth about Markets*, London: Penguin Books, 2003.

Commandment One: Quit Taking Risks

1 Colman, K., 'Health and Health Services: changes over the last seven years', *Health Trends* 1998, 30(1) 5-7.

2 Wanless, D., *Securing our Future Health: taking a long-term view: an interim report*, London: HM Treasury, 2001, p. 164; House of Commons Health Committee, *The Use of New Medical Technologies within the NHS*, London: TSO, 2005; Cooksey, D. *A Review of UK Health Research Funding*, London: HM Treasury, 2006, p. 35.

3 McClellan, M., Kessler, A. *et al.*, 'Technological Change Around the World: evidence from heart attack care', TECH, *Health Affairs*, May/June 2001:25-42.

4 Fitzpatrick, A., 'The Cutting Edge', *Medical Technology and Innovation*, MTG, Issue 14, 2007.

5 Packer, C. *et al.*, 'International Diffusion of New Health Technologies: a ten-country analysis of six health technologies', *International Journal of Technology Assessment in Healthcare*, Cambridge University Press, Issue 22, pp. 419-428, 2006.

6 National Radiotherapy Advisory Group, *Radiotherapy: developing a world class service for England*, London: NRAG, 2007, p. 14.

7 OECD, *OECD Health Data*, Paris: OECD, 2008.

8 House of Commons Health Committee, *The Use of New Medical Technologies within the NHS*, London: TSO, 2005, Ev 65, The Medical Technology Group.

9 Fuchs, V., 'Healthcare expenditures re-examined', *Ann Intern Med.* 2005;143:76-78

10 Debnath, D., 'Activity analysis of telemedicine in the UK', *Postgrad. Med. J.* 2004;80;335-338

11 Christensen, C., Bohmer, R. and Kenagy, J., 'Will Disruptive Innovations Cure Healthcare?', *HBR*, September–October 2000.

12 Barlow, J. and Burn, J., *All Change Please: putting the best new healthcare ideas into practice*, London: Policy Exchange, 2008, ch. 2.

13 www.bbbc.org.uk

14 Mawson, A., *The Social Entrepreneur: making communities work*, London: Atlantic Books, 2008, p. 90.

15 Tallis, R., *Hippocratic Oaths: medicine and its discontents*, London: Atlantic Books, 2004, p. 82.

16 Office of Government & Commerce, *Change Capability Review*, London: TSO, 2006.

17 See:
http://www.channel4.com/news/articles/dispatches/liam+halligan+investigates+operation+delays/267683

18 NHS Confederation, *The Challenges of Leadership in the NHS*, London: NHS Confederation, 2007, p. 5.

19 Stanton, P., 'Paul Stanton on local legitimacy in the NHS', *HSJ*, 27 June 2008;
http://www.hsj.co.uk/acutecare/opinion/2008/06/paul_stanton_on_national_politicisation_and_local_democratic.html

20 Burnham, A., 'The People Project', *Guardian*, 16 January 2008;
http://www.guardian.co.uk/commentisfree/2008/jan/16/politics.publicservices

21 Monitor, *Review of NHS foundation trusts' annual plans 2008/09*, London: Monitor, 2008, p. 6.

22 Greenhalgh, T. *et al.*, 'Diffusion of Innovations in Service Organizations: systematic review and recommendations', *The Milbank Quarterly*, Issue 82, pp. 581-629, 2004.

23 Bate, P., Mendelm P. and Robert, G., *Organizing for Quality: the improvement journeys of leading hospitals in Europe and the United States*, Oxford: Radcliffe, 2008.

24 Ferlie, E. and Shortell, S., 'Improving the Quality of Health Care in the United Kingdom and the United States: A Framework for Change', *The Milbank Quarterly*, Vol. 79, No. 2, 2001.

NOTES

Commandment Two: Be Inflexible

1   Greener, I., 'Where are the medical voices raised in protest?', *BMJ* 2006;333:660

2   Watkin, B., *The National Health Service: the first phase 1948-1974 and after*, London: George Allen & Unwin, 1978, p. 40.

3   http://news.bbc.co.uk/1/hi/uk_politics/6752975.stm

4   Hall, E., Propper, C. and Van Reenen, J., *Can Pay Regulation Kill? Panel Data Evidence on the Effect of Labor Markets on Hospital Performance*, CEP Discussion Paper No 843, 2008.

5   House of Commons Health Committee, Health Inequalities: Third Report of Session 2008-09, London: TSO, 2009, HI 129: Professor Peter Smith.

6   Field, S., Smith, S., Bernath, O. and Roland, M., 'Polyclinics: an integrating or disintegrating force?' Debate hosted by Civitas at The Royal College of Surgeons of England, 29 May 2008; http://www.civitas.org.uk/nhs/download/polyclinics_29May.pdf

7   *Hansard*, 24 April 2007: column 808; http://www.publications.parliament.uk/pa/cm200607/cmhansrd/cm070424/debtext/70424-0006.htm

8   Department of Health, *The Operating Framework for the NHS in England, 2009/10*, London: TSO, 2008, ch. 4.

9   Barker, R, 'Richard Barker on why the IT programme is never going to come right', *HSJ*, 16 November 2006.

10 House of Commons Committee of Public Accounts, *Department of Health: the national programme for IT in the NHS*, London: TSO, 2006.

11 Randell, B., 'A computer scientist's reactions to NPfIT', *Journal of Information Technology* 2007; 22, 222–234.

12 Timmins, N., 'Health records scheme at "pivotal" point', *The Financial Times,* 12 December 2008.

13 Goldman, M., 'Mark Goldman on becoming an NHS follower ', *HSJ,* 10 March 2009.

14 Newdick, C., *Who Should We Treat? Rights, Rationing and Resources in the NHS* (2nd edn), Oxford: Oxford University Press, 2005, pp. 206-11.

15 Christie, S., 'Sophie Christie on the Lucentis drug controversy', *HSJ*, 14 February 2008.

16 Leatherman, S. and Sutherland, K., *The Quest for Quality: refining the NHS reforms*, London: The Nuffield Trust, 2008, ch. 2.

17 Darzi, A., *High Quality Care for All: NHS next stage review final report*, London: TSO, 2008; Light, D., Analysis: 'Will the NHS strategic plan benefit patients?', *BMJ* 2008;337:a824

18 NHS Confederation, *From the Ground Up: how autonomy could deliver a better NHS*, London: NHS Confederation, 2007.

Commandment Three: Isolate Yourself

1 Gleave, R., *Across the Pond—lessons from the US on integrated healthcare*, London: The Nuffield Trust, 2009.

2 Garlick, A. and Fagin, L., 'The doctor-manager relationship', *Advances in Psychiatric Treatment*, Vol. 11, 2005, pp. 241–252.

3 Dixon, J., Chantler, C. and Billings, J., 'Competition on Outcomes and Physician Leadership Are Not Enough to Reform Health Care', *JAMA* 2007;298(12):1445-1447

4 Preston, C. *et al.*, 'Left in limbo: patients' views on care across the primary-secondary care interface', *Qual. Health Care* 1999;8;16-21

5 Cowie, L. *et al.*, 'Experience of continuity of care of patients with multiple long-term conditions in England', *J Health Serv Res Policy* 2009;14:82-87.

6 Cowie *et al.*, 'Experience of continuity of care of patients with multiple long-term conditions in England', 2009.

7 Cited in Carlisle, D., 'Lost for words', *HSJ*, 29 January 2009, pp. 18-20.

8 Davies, P., 'The great NHS communication breakdown', *BMJ* 2008;337:a664 (published 4 July 2008).

9 http://www.nchod.nhs.uk/

10 Cited in Gleave, R., *Across the Pond—lessons from the US on integrated healthcare*, London: The Nuffield Trust, 2009, p. 10.

11 Forrest, C.B., Glade, G.B., Baker, A.E. *et al.* 'Coordination of specialty referrals and physician satisfaction with referral care', *Arch Pediatr Adolesc Med* 2000; 154(5): 499-506.

12 Ham, C., *Integrating NHS Care: lessons from the frontline*, London: The Nuffield Trust, 2008; Davies, P., *Local Hospitals: lessons for the NHS, Central Middlesex Hospital Case Study*, London: NHS Confederation, 2009.

13 Gleave, *Across the Pond*, 2009.

14 Gleave, *Across the Pond*, 2009; Light D. and Dixon, M., 'Making the NHS more like Kaiser Permanente', *BMJ* 2004;328: 763-5; Feachem, R.G.A. and Sekhri, N.K., 'Moving towards true integration', *BMJ* 2005;330: 787-8

15 Feachem, R., Sekhri, N. and White, K., 'Getting more for their dollar: a comparison of the NHS with California's Kaiser Permanente', *BMJ* 2002;324: 135-41.

16 Royal College of Physicians, *Teams without Walls: the value of medical innovation and leadership*, London: RCP, 2008.

17 Davies, *Local Hospitals: lessons for the NHS, Central Middlesex Hospital Case Study.*

18 Healthcare Commission, *Listening, Learning and Working Together? A national study of how well healthcare organisations engage local people in planning and improving their services*, London: Healthcare Commission, 2009.

19 Davies, *Local Hospitals: lessons for the NHS, Central Middlesex Hospital Case Study.* .

20 Cowie, *et al.*, 'Experience of continuity of care of patients with multiple long-term conditions in England', 2009.

Commandment Four: Assume Infallibility

1   Prochaska, F.K., *Philanthropy and the Hospitals of London*, Oxford: Clarendon Press, 1992, p. 130.

2   http://www.number10.gov.uk/Page16283

3   *Hansard*, 3 July 2008: Column 1129; http://www.publications.parliament.uk/pa/cm200708/cmhansrd/cm 080703/debtext/80703-0020.htm#08070352004169

4   http://news.bbc.co.uk/1/hi/health/7475561.stm

5   Nolte, E. and McKee, M., 'Measuring the health of nations: updating an earlier analysis', *Health Affairs*, 2008, 27(1):58-71

6   Verdecchia, A. *et al.*, 'Recent cancer survival in Europe: a 2000-02 period analysis of EUROCARE-4 data', *Lancet Oncol*, 2007 doi: 10.1016/S0140-6736(08)61345-8.

7   Rachet, B. *et al.*, 'Population-based cancer survival trends in England and Wales up to 2007: an assessment of the NHS cancer plan for England', *Lancet Oncol*, doi:10.1016/S1470-2045(09)70028-2.

8   Gubb, J., *Just How Well Are We? A glance at trends in avoidable mortality from cancer and circulatory disease in England & Wales*, London: Civitas, 2007.

9   Grieve, R., Hutton, J., Bhalla, A., Rastenytë, D., Ryglewicz, D., Sarti, C. *et al.*, 'A comparison of the costs and survival of hospital-admitted stroke patients across Europe', *Stroke*, 2001;32:1684-91; Weir, N.U., Sandercock, P.A., Lewis, S.C., Signorini, D.F., Warlow, C.P., 'Variations between countries in outcome after stroke in the International Stroke Trial (IST)', *Stroke*, 2001;32;1370-7; Gray, L.J., Sprigg, N., Bath, P.M., Sorensen, P., Lindenstrom, E., Boysen, G. *et al.*, 'Significant variation in mortality and functional outcome after acute ischaemic stroke between Western countries: data from the tinzaparin in acute ischaemic stroke trial (TAIST)', *J Neurol Neurosurg Psychiatry*, 2006;77:327-33, cited in Markus, H., 'Improving the outcome of stroke: UK needs to reorganise services to follow the example of other countries', *BMJ* 2007;335:359-360.

10 Weir *et al.*, 'Variations between countries in outcome after stroke in the International Stroke Trial (IST)', *Stroke* 2001;32;1370-7

11 Bosanquet, N. *et al.*, *Making the NHS the Best Insurance Policy in the World*, London: Reform, 2008, p. 11. These measures are, of course, subject to a number of factors outside the immediate scope of any health system, such as poverty, housing, unemployment and social mobility.

12 Health Consumer Powerhouse, *Euro Health Consumer Index 2008*, Stockholm: Health Consumer Powerhouse, 2008.

13 Richards, N. and Coulter, A., *Is the NHS Becoming More Patient-centred? Trends from the national surveys of NHS patients in England 2002-2007*, Oxford: The Picker Institute, 2007.

14 For a discussion around this see: Gubb, 'Just how well are we?'.

15 Seddon, N., *Quite Like Heaven? Options for the NHS in a consumer age*, London: Civitas, 2007; Gubb, J., 'Why the NHS is the sick man of Europe', *Civitas Rev* 2008;5:1.

16 Green, D., and Irvine, B., 'Social insurance: the right way forward for health care in the United Kingdom', *BMJ* 2002;325:488-490

17 Mossialos, E., and Le Grand, J., *Health Care and Cost Containment in the European Union*, Aldershot: Ashgate Press, 1999.

18 http://www.number10.gov.uk/Page14171

19 See, for example: Elledge, J., 'Primary care czar accuses GPs of whinging', *Healthcare Republic*, 1 October 2008; http://www.healthcarerepublic.com/news/GP/LatestNews/850093/Primary-care-czar-accuses-GPs-whinging/?CMP=EMC-DAILYNEWS

20 Coates, S., 'Lib Dems call for drunks to face A&E treatment charges', *The Times*, 14 September 2007.

21 Rogers, H., Maher, L. and Plsek, P., 'Better by design: using simple rules to improve access to secondary care', *BMJ* 2008;337:a2321

Commandment Five: Play Game Close to Foul Line

1   Keough, D., *The Ten Commandments for Business Failure*, New York: Penguin Books, 2008, p. 68.

2   Halligan, A., 'The importance of values in healthcare', *J R Soc Med* 2008;101:480-481.

3   Klein, R., 'The new model NHS: performance, perceptions and expectations, *British Medical Bulletin*, doi:10.1093/bmb/ldm013

4   Department of Health, *Our Healthier Nation: a contract for health*, London: TSO, 1998.

5   Healthcare Commission, *The Annual Health Check 2007/08*, London: Healthcare Commission, 2008, Annex A-C.

6   http://www.qof.ic.nhs.uk/

7   O'Neill, O., *A Question of Trust*, Cambridge: Cambridge University Press, 2002.

8   Gubb, J. and Li, G., *Checking-up on Doctors: a review of the quality and outcomes framework for general practitioners*, London: Civitas, 2008.

9   Gubb, J., *Why Are We Waiting? An analysis of waiting times in the NHS*, London: Civitas, 2008.

10 Gubb, J., *The NHS and the NHS Plan: Is the extra money working'*, London: Civitas, 2006.

11 See: http://www.hpa.org.uk/webw/HPAweb&Page&HPAwebAutoListName/Page/1191942126522?p=1191942126522

12 Royal Statistical Society Working Party on Performance Monitoring in the Public Service, *Performance Indicators: Good, Bad and Ugly*, London: RSA, 2004.

13 Harrison, A. and Thorlby, R., *The 18-week Waiting Times Target*, London: The King's Fund, 2007, p. 3.

14 Seddon, J., *Systems Thinking in the Public Sector: the failure of the reform regime . . . and a manifesto for a better way*, Axminster: Triarchy Press, 2008.

15 Department of Health, Hospital Activity Statistics, 2008;
    http://www.performance.doh.gov.uk/hospitalactivity/data_request
    s/total_time_ae.htm

16 Mayhew, L. and Smith, D., 'Using queuing theory to analyse the
    Government's 4-h completion target in Accident and Emergency
    departments', *Health Care Manage Sci* 2008 11:11–21.

17 BMA Survey of Accident and Emergency Waiting Times, 2005
    http://www.bma.org.uk/ap.nsf/Content/AESurveyReport310106~in
    troduction?OpenDocument&Highlight=2,A&E,survey

18 Mayhew and Smith, 'Using queuing theory to analyse the
    Government's 4-h completion target in Accident and Emergency
    departments', *Health Care Manage Sci* 2008 11:11–21; Gubb, *Why Are
    We Waiting?* pp. 10-15; Bevan, G. and Hood, C., 'Have targets
    improved performance in the English NHS?', *BMJ* 2006 332: 419-
    422; Campbell, D., 'Scandal of patients left for hours outside A&E',
    Observer, 17 February 2008.

19 Gubb, *Why Are We Waiting?*, 2008.

20 Orendi, J., 'Health-care organisation, hospital-bed occupancy, and
    MRSA', *Lancet* 2008 26;371(9622):1401-2.

21 Healthcare Commission, *Patient Survey 2005 — PCTs*, London: TSO,
    2005, Executive Summary.

22 Gubb and Li, *Checking-up on Doctors*, 2009.

23 West, D., 'Eight minute target holds back service improvement',
    HSJ, 4 December 2008.

24 Berwick, D., 'A primer on leading the improvement of systems',
    BMJ 1996;312:619-622. In one survey by the BMA, only 26 per cent
    of A&E staff view figures submitted by their department as a fair
    reflection of performance;
    http://www.bma.org.uk/ap.nsf/Content/AESurveyReport310106~in
    troduction?OpenDocument&Highlight=2,A&E,survey

25 Gubb and Li, *Checking-up on Doctors*; Goodrich, J. and Cornwell, J.,
    Seeing the Person in the Patient: The Point of Care Review Paper,
    London: The King's Fund, 2008.

26 Jones, D. and Mitchell, A., *Lean Thinking for the NHS*, London: NHS
    Confederation, 2006.

27 Youngson, R., *Compassion in healthcare: the missing dimension of
    healthcare reform?*, London: NHS Confederation, 2008; Halligan, A.,
    'The first casualty of NHS reform — lost NHS values', *Br J Healthcare
    Manage* 2007 13(8):288-290; Gubb and Li, *Checking-up on Doctors*,
    ch. 4.

Commandment Six: Don't Take Time to Think

1 Bate, P., Mendel, P. and Robert, G., *Organizing for Quality: the
   improvement journeys of leading hospitals in Europe and the United
   States*. Oxford: Radcliffe, 2008.

2 Bate, Mendel and Robert, *Organizing for Quality*, 2008.

3 Bate, Mendel and Robert, *Organizing for Quality*, 2008, Foreword.

4 Webster, C., *The NHS: A Political History* (2nd edn), Oxford: Oxford
   University Press, 2002; Klein, R., *The New Politics of the NHS: from
   creation to reinvention* (5th edn), Oxford: Radcliffe Medical
   Publishing, 2006.

5 Davies, P., 'Between Health and Illness', *Perspectives in Biology and
   Medicine* 50:3 444-452, 2007.

6 Edwards, N., 'The questions to ask yourself about policy', *HSJ*, 12
   June 2008, pp. 18-19.

7 Mulholland, H., 'Brown: NHS renewal is biggest priority',
   Guardian, 7 January 2008.

8 Light, D., 'Will the NHS strategic plan benefit patients?', *BMJ*
   2008;337:a824.

9 House of Commons Health Committee, *NHS Next Stage Review:
   First Report of Session 2008–09*, Vol. I, London: TSO, 2009.

10 Blackler, F., 'Chief Executives and the Modernization of the English
    National Health Service', *Leadership*, Vol. 2, No. 1, 2006, pp. 5-30.

11 Royal Society for the Encouragement of Arts, Manufactures and Commerce, *Corporate Governance in the Public and Voluntary Sectors,* London: RSA, 2002.

12 Audit Commission, *Auditor's Local Evaluation 2007/08,* London: TSO, 2008.

13 Cochrane, A.L., *Effectiveness and Efficiency,* London: Nuffield Provincial Hospitals Trust, 1972.

14 NHS Confederation, *Disruptive Innovation: what does it mean for the NHS?,* London: NHS Confederation, 2008, p. 6.

15 Liker, J.K., *The Toyota Way: 14 management principles,* New York: McGraw-Hill, 2004.

16 Young, T. and McClean, S., 'A critical look at Lean Thinking in healthcare', *Qual Saf Health Care* 2008;17:382-386; Jones, D. and Mitchell, A., *Lean Thinking for the NHS,* London: NHS Confederation, 2006.

17 Haynes, A. *et al.,* 'A surgical safety checklist to reduce morbidity and mortality in a global population, *N Engl J Med* 360;5, 2009.

18 Perlin, J. *et al.,* 'The veterans health administration: quality, value, accountability and information as transforming strategies for patient-centred care', *Am J Managed Care* 2004;10:828-36.

19 Boaden, R., Quality improvement: theory and practice, *Br J Healthcare Manage,* Vol. 15, No 1, 2009, pp. 12-16.

20 Bate, Mendel and Robert, *Organizing for Quality,* 2008.

21 Mechanic, D., 'How should hamsters run? Some observations about sufficient patient time in primary care', *BMJ* Aug 2001; 323: 266-268.

Commandment Seven: Put Faith in Consultants

1 Cited in Towill, D., 'Leadership in the NHS: what can the Department of Health learn from Gerry Robinson—the programme?', *Leadership in Health Services,* Vol. 21, No. 3, 2008, pp. 151-57.

2 CHKS, '48 CHKS clients achieve "excellent" in Healthcare Commission rating', Press Release, 2008; http://www.chks.co.uk/index.php?id=542

3 Bate, P., Mendel, P. and Robert, G., *Organizing for Quality: the improvement journeys of leading hospitals in Europe and the United States*, Oxford: Radcliffe, 2008.

4 Reed, K., 'NHS becomes fourth largest consulting market', *Accountancy Age*, 29 September 2006.

5 Charter, D., 'Stop management consultancy waste', *The Times*, 8 June 2006.

6 Reed, 'NHS becomes fourth largest consulting market', 2006.

7 National Audit Office, *Department of Health: The Paddington Health Campus scheme*, London: TSO, 2006; National Audit Office, *Good Practice Briefing for PFI/PPP*, London: TSO, 2006.

8 Department of Health, Press Release: 'Hewitt announces action to turnaround NHS finances', 25 January 2005.

9 House of Commons Health Committee, *NHS Deficits: First Report of Session 2006–07*, London: TSO, 2006, Uncorrected transcript of oral evidence taken before the Health Committee 23 November 2006, HC 94–i, Q89.

10 House of Commons Health Committee, *NHS Deficits: First Report of Session 2006–07*, London: TSO, 2006, pp. 49-51.

11 *Hansard*, 17 Dec 2007 : Column 1217W (NHS Trusts: Finance); http://www.publications.parliament.uk/pa/cm200708/cmhansrd/cm071217/text/71217w0064.htm#07121884000720

12 Healthcare Commission, *The Annual Health Check 2007/08*, London: Healthcare Commission, 2008.

13 Healthcare Commission, *Annual health check 2007/08 — Performance of Surrey and Sussex Healthcare NHS Trust*, London: Healthcare Commission, 2008.

14 See:
http://www.dh.gov.uk/en/Publicationsandstatistics/Publications/Pu
blicationsPolicyAndGuidance/DH_065818

15 Mooney, H., 'HSJ commissioning supplement: an in-depth look at FESC', *HSJ*, 1 November 2008.

16 Lithgow, T., 'Doubts emerge over value for money of private firm scheme', *Pulse*, 13 August 2008.

17 Gainsbury, S., 'FESC is thrown open without Treasury probe', *HSJ*, 13 March 2008.

18 Fish, D., Marshall, M., Simpson, J. and Ribeiro, B., 'Clinical leadership: lost or at a new dawn?', Debate hosted by Civitas at the House of Commons, 26 November 2008;
http://www.civitas.org.uk/nhs/download/clinical_leadership.pdf

19 Towill, 'Leadership in the NHS', 2008.

Commandment Eight: Love Your Bureaucracy

1 Department of Health, *The New NHS: modern, dependable,*, London: TSO, 1997.

2 Gershon, P., *Releasing Resources to the Front Line: independent review of public sector efficiency*, London: HMSO, 2004, pp. 34, 52.

3 Department of Health, *Reconfiguring the Department of Health's Arm's Length Bodies*, London: TSO, 2004.

4 Department of Health, *The NHS Improvement Plan: Putting people at the heart of public services,* London: TSO, 2004.

5 Darzi, A., *High Quality Care for All: NHS next stage review final report*, London: TSO, 2008, p. 30.

6 Walshe, K., 'The rise of regulation in the NHS', *BMJ* 2002;324:967-70.

7 Department of Health, *Review of NHS Data Collections 2005: report for the Department of Health and NHS Health and Social Care Information Centre*, London: TSO, 2006.

8   NHS Confederation, *The bureaucratic burden in the NHS,* London: The NHS Confederation, 2007; Blunden, F., 'Frances Blunden on waste and bureaucracy', *HSJ,* 23 April 2009.

9   Department of Health, *Review of NHS Data Collections 2005,* 2006.

10   NHS Confederation, *The Bureaucratic Burden in the NHS,* London: The NHS Confederation, 2007, Annex A; Walshe, 'The rise of regulation in the NHS'.

11   http://www.crhp.org.uk/

12   Blunden, 'Frances Blunden on waste and bureaucracy', 2009.

13   Tallis, R., *Hippocratic Oaths: medicine and its discontents,* London: Atlantic Books, 2004, p. 87.

14   DH Press Release, (DH) 'Government outlines changes to GP quality incentive scheme', 19 March 2009.

15   Santry, C., 'Health watchdog handover is on 'red risk', *HSJ,* 5 February 2009.

16   NHS Confederation, *The Bureaucratic Burden in the NHS,* 2007, p. 2.

17   NHS Confederation, *Briefing 92: Smarter Reporting,* London: NHS Confederation, 2003.

18   The Information Centre, *Staff in the NHS 1997-2007 (England),* London: The Information Centre, 2008; http://www.ic.nhs.uk/webfiles/publications/nhsstaff2007/Staff%20i n%20the%20NHS%20leaflet.pdf

19   House of Commons Health Committee, *Department of Health Written Evidence to the Committee,* London: TSO, 2005, HC 736-111, Table 3.7.1.

20   Donnelly, L., 'NHS bureaucracy spending doubles', *Sunday Telegraph,* 11 April 2009.

21   Tallis, *Hippocratic Oaths,* 2004, pp. 85-86.

22   Keough, D., *The Ten Commandments for Business Failure,* New York: Penguin Books, 2008, p. 126.

Commandment Nine: Send Mixed Messages

1   See:
    http://money.cnn.com/galleries/2008/fortune/0803/gallery.people
    management.fortune/3.html

2   Martinez, M., 'Disney training works magic - Walt Disney
    Productions - HR Agenda: Training and Development', *HR
    Magazine*, May 1992.

3   Lynch, L., 'Sustaining innovation: Walt Disney instilled how',
    Training & Development, June 2001.

4   Halligan, A., Fish, D., Simpson, J., Marshall, M. and Ribeiro, B.,
    'Clinical leadership: lost or at a new dawn?', Debate hosted by
    Civitas at The House of Commons, 26 November 2008;
    http://www.civitas.org.uk/nhs/download/clinical_leadership.pdf

5   Boaden, R., 'Quality Improvement: Theory and Practice', *Br J
    Healthcare Manage*, Vol. 15, No. 1, 2009, pp. 12-16.

6   Bate, P., Mendel, P. and Robert, G., *Organizing for Quality: The
    improvement journeys of leading hospitals in Europe and the United
    States*, Oxford: Radcliffe, 2008, p. 200.

7   http://www.griffinhealth.org/AboutGriffin/Mission.aspx
    Its mission statement reads: "Griffin Hospital is committed to
    providing personalized, humanistic, consumer-driven health care
    in a healing environment, to empowering individuals to be actively
    involved in decisions affecting their care and well-being through
    access to information and education, and to providing leadership
    to improve the health of the community we serve."

8   Capodagli, B. and Jackson, L., *The Disney Way: Harnessing the
    Management Secrets of Disney in your Company*, (2nd edn), New
    York: McGraw-Hill Professional, 2006, pp. 32-34.

9   Bate, Mendel and Robert, *Organizing for Quality*, 2008, ch. 3.

10 Bate, Mendel and Robert, *Organizing for Quality*, 2008, p. 52.

11 Healthcare Commission, *National NHS Staff Survey 2008: summary of
    key findings*, London: Healthcare Commission, 2008.

12   Department of Health, *NHS Operating Framework for 2009/10*, London: TSO, 2008, pp. 23-4.

13   Department of Health, *NHS Operating Framework for 2009/10*, 2008, p. 24.

14   Maynard, A., 'Alan Maynard on Incentivising Quality', *HSJ Intelligence*, 27 November 2008.

15   Harvey, S., Liddell, A. and McMahon, L., *Windmill 2007: the future of healthcare reforms in England*, London: The King's Fund, 2007, p. 1.

16   Dixon, A., *Quality in a Cold Climate: is the NHS on course?*, The King's Fund monthly update, December 2008; http://www.kingsfund.org.uk/publications/articles/quality_in_a_co ld.html
     Indeed, the purpose of even having a one-year Operating Framework is not at all clear in a 'locally driven [NHS], looking outwards not upwards', where commissioners are encouraged to 'take a long-term view of population health and changing requirements'.

17   Harvey, Liddell and McMahon, *Windmill 2007*, 2007, p. 1.

18   Healthcare Commission, *Learning from Investigations*, London: Healthcare Commission, 2008.

Commandment Ten: Be Afraid of the Future

1   Tallis, R., *Hippocratic Oaths: medicine and its discontents*, London: Atlantic Books, 2004, ch. 8.

2   Christensen, C., Bohmer, R. and Kenagy, J., 'Will Disruptive Innovations Cure Healthcare?', *HBR*, September–October 2000.

3   Lomas, J., 'Health Services Research: More lessons from Kaiser Permanente and Veterans' Affairs healthcare system', *BMJ* 2003;327;1301-1302.

4   Sikora, K., 'Paying for cancer care—a new dilemma', *J R Soc Med* 2007;100:166–169.

5   Tallis, *Hippocratic Oaths,* 2004, ch. 2.

6 Tallis, *Hippocratic Oaths,* 2004, ch. 8.

7 Christensen, Bohmer and Kenagy, 'Will Disruptive Innovations Cure Healthcare?'2000.

8 Gubb, J., 'Should patients be able to pay top-up fees to receive the treatment they want? Yes', *BMJ* 2008;336:1104.

9 Leatherman, S. and Sutherland, K., *The Quest for Quality: refining the NHS reforms,* London: The Nuffield Trust, 2008, p. 17.

10 Blackler, F., 'Chief Executives and the Modernization of the English National Health Service', *Leadership,* Vol. 2, No. 1, 2006, pp. 5-30; Harvey, S., Liddell, A. and McMahon, L., *Windmill 2007: the future of healthcare reforms in England,* London: The King's Fund, 2007; NHS Confederation, *The Challenges of Leadership in the NHS,* London: NHS Confederation, 2007.

11 Tallis, *Hippocratic Oaths,* 2004; Halligan, A., 'The first casualty of NHS reform—lost NHS values', *Br J Healthcare Manage* 2007 13(8):288-290.

12 IOM, in Khon, L.T., Corrigan, J.M. and Donaldson, M.S. (eds), *To Err is Human: building a safer healthcare system,* Washington DC: The National Academies Press, 1999; IOM, *Crossing the Quality Chasm: a new health system for the twenty-first century,* Washington DC: The National Academies Press, 2001; Canadian Health Services Research Foundation, 'Myth: we can improve quality one doctor at a time', *Eurohealth* 2008;14:37-8; Taylor-Adams, S. and Vincent, C., *Systems Analysis of Clinical Incidents: the London protocol,* London: Imperial College London, 2004.

13 Howie, J.G.R., 'Addressing the credibility gap in general practice research: better theory; more feeling; less strategy', *Br J Gen Pract,* 1996, 46;479-487.

14 Britnell, M., Farrar, M., Richardson, T. and Dixon, M., 'Commission impossible: is world class commissioning achievable in the NHS?', debate hosted by Civitas at The House of Commons, 16 July 2008; www.civitas.org.uk/nhs/download/wcc_16July.pdf

15 Tallis, *Hippocratic Oaths*, 2004, pp. 139-66; Christensen, C., Bohmer, R. and Kenagy, J., 'Will disruptive innovations cure healthcare?', *HBR*, September–October 2000.

16 Darling, M., Parry, C. and Moore, J., 'Learning in the thick of it', *HBR* July-August 2005, pp. 1-9.

17 Reynard, J. and Biers, S., *Oxford Handbook of Urology*, Oxford: OUP, 2006, p. 6.

18 Christensen, Bohmer and Kenagy, 'Will disruptive innovations cure healthcare?', 2000.

19 Healthcare Commission, *National NHS Staff Survey 2008: summary of key findings*, London: Healthcare Commission, 2008.

Commandment Eleven: Lose Passion for Work and Life

1   Smith J., Walshe K. and Hunter D.J., 'The "redisorganisation" of the NHS', *BMJ* 2001;323:1262-3.

2   Maynard, A., 'Keeping up with the Joneses', in Appleby, J. (ed.), *Funding Health Care: 2008 and Beyond*, London: King's Fund, 2006, p. 19.

3   Klein, R., 'The New Model NHS: performance, perceptions and expectations', *British Medical Bulletin*, 2007; 1-12.

4   Tallis, R., *Hippocratic Oaths: Medicine and its Discontents*, London: Atlantic Books, 2004, pp. 210-16.

5   Healthcare Commission, *Acute Trusts: the views of staff*, London: Healthcare Commission, 2006, p. 2; Royal College of Nurses, *At Breaking Point? A survey of wellbeing and working lives of nurses in 2005*, London: RCN, 2006; Healthcare Commission, *Ward Staffing*, London: Healthcare Commission, 2005.

6   Davies, P., 'The ups and downs of GP life', *Br J Gen Pract.*, 2008; 58(546): 53.

7   Smith, R., 'Why are doctors so unhappy? There are probably many causes, some of them deep', *BMJ* 2001 May 5; 322(7294).

8   Godlee, F., 'While Rome burns', *BMJ*, 2006; 333; 7569, editorial.

9   See, for instance: 'Cleanliness inspector in every hospital', *The Times*, 10 September 2007; http://www.timesonline.co.uk/tol/news/uk/health/article2049252.ece

10 Paddock, C., 'Most British doctors would no longer recommend a career in medicine, *Medical News Today*, 12 April 2007; http://www.medicalnewstoday.com/articles/67662.php

11 Healthcare Commission, *National NHS staff survey 2006*, London: Healthcare Commission, 2007.

12 Healthcare Commission. *National Survey of NHS Staff 2007*, Healthcare Commission, 2008.

13 Healthcare Commission, *National NHS Staff Survey 2008: summary of key findings*, London: Healthcare Commission, 2008.

14 Godlee, F., 'Doctors' health matters', *BMJ* 2008;337:a2527; Brewster, J.M., 'Doctors' health', *BMJ* 2008;337:a2161 7 November 2008.

15 Frank E., 'Physician health and patient care', *JAMA* 2004;291:637.

16 Tallis, *Hippocratic Oaths*, 2004, p. 211.

Conclusion

1   O'Neill, O., *A Question of Trust*, Cambridge: Cambridge University Press, 2002.

2   Davies, P., *Local Hospitals: lessons for the NHS, Central Middlesex Hospital case study*, London: NHS Confederation, 2009.

3   http://www.ucl.ac.uk/news/news-articles/0811/08111705

4   See: http://www.drfosterintelligence.co.uk/successStories/detail.asp?caseID=patientExperience4

5   Davies, P., The Beleaguered Consultation, *Br J Gen Pract.*, 2006 March 1; 56(524): 226–229.

6   Cocksedge, S., *Listening as Work in Primary Care*, Oxford: Radcliffe Publishing Ltd, 2005.

7   Berwick, D., Foreword in Bate, P., Mendel, P. and Robert, G.,
    *Organizing for Quality: the improvement journeys of leading hospitals in
    Europe and the United States*, Oxford: Radcliffe, 2008.

8   Cited in Mawson, A., *The Social Entrepreneur: making communities
    work*, London: Atlantic Books, 2008, p. 155.

9   Patel, A. and Ingleton, R., 'Apple's way will bear most fruit', *HSJ*,
    15 January 2009, p. 16.

10 Tudor-Hart, J., *A New Kind of Doctor: the General Practitioner's part in
    the health of the community*, London: Merlin Press, 1988.